SEX POSITIONS

Tips and tricks to increase intimacy and desire in sexual performance to have a better sex life. A step by step guide to hot sex in bed, in bathrooms, in car, outdoor and everywhere.

DONNA DARE

Table of Contents

Description

Sexual positions can add a whole new realm of pleasure and help you see your partner in a whole new way. These different positions allow you to view your partner from all angles of intercourse, which for men, can be highly arousing because men are mainly visual when it comes to sexual arousal.

Not changing up sexual positions can cause love lives to become stagnant and redundant and can ultimately lead to betrayal and individuals going astray in their relationships. Relationships and sex lives can be spiced up easily by the introduction of new sex positions, and they should be introduced whenever possible. Along with other types of experimentations and stimulations. Whatever you will gain from this book, I hope it will be a mixture of arousal, interest, and excitement. Deciding to take a hold of your love and sex life and change up things is a huge step in the right direction. Most people stay in their comfort zone because they think it is comfortable – when it really is not. Wouldn't you be more comfortable in your relationship and sex life if you were both getting out of it what you wanted instead of compromising and not trying anything new?

This guide will focus on the following:

- Easy Tips to Make Her Hornier
- Spicing up your sex life
- 17 Sexual and Aphrodisiacs Food
- 5 Shocking Things That Can Help You Last Longer in Bed
- Different Types of Sexual Play
- Playing in Public
- Flexibility Positions
- Relaxing Positions
- Superior Sex Positions
- Sensual Positions
- Sex for People with Mobility Challenges... AND MORE!!!

Introduction

Sex is such an interesting part of our lives. We can become completely different people once we sneak under the sheets with someone. There is so much to explore, so many parts of our human psyche that are still untapped, waiting for the right key to come unlock them. I believe that almost anyone can be consumed by the allure sex poses. It becomes a challenge to reach certain milestones – losing your virginity, receiving your first oral sex, giving your first oral sex, having sex in public for the first time, trying your first sex toy, making love for the first time. It's fun. There's also a certain amount of ego involved. It feels good to be doing this stuff, and I do think that sex is a fundamental need we have as human beings.

But it's also important not to place too much emphasis on your "success" or "failure" in this conquest. I have been through periods where I was not having any sex, and for whatever reason, I let it affect my self-esteem and my sense of self-worth. This is an unhealthy view of sexuality. You are letting your mind become vulnerable to an outside force that can be largely out of your control. The conquest should not be a conquest at all. There should not be anything to conquer, or to do better than someone else, or to do before someone else.

It should be an exploration of this aspect of life. You should try your best to seek the truth in your sex life. Find out what you truly want. Find a partner or partners who share your desires. Make the most of those experiences. Don't do this for personal gain or to make yourself feel better. Don't do it to selfishly "get yourself off."

Do it to genuinely share a unique connection with someone.

Do it to have the most fun you possibly can.

I mean, that's what this is all about right? Having a good time?

So, take what you have learned here, go forth in your sex life with confidence and determination to find that truth which only you can find, and I will leave you with one last thing:

This may be **The Guide to Great Sex**, but in reality, you are your own guide to great sex.

Navigate wisely.

Chapter 1: Easy Tips to Make Her Hornier

A standout amongst the most successive protestations men have about their spouses is that they wish their ladies would start sex all the more frequently, or if nothing else that they would be more receptive to their sexual suggestions. The explanation behind this basic inconsistency is that male sexual yearning is heartier and more unconstrained, while female sexual craving is more variable and receptive to the earth.

With regards to sex, men are for the most part genitally centered, while for ladies, sex is a full psyche and body experience. The fundamental clash between men furthermore, ladies, sexually, is that men are similar to firefighters, and ladies are similar to flame. To men, sex is a crisis, and regardless of what they're doing, they can be prepared in two minutes. Ladies, then again, are similar to flame. They're extremely energizing, yet the conditions have to be precisely a good fit for it to happen.

For women to want sex it has to be sex worth having.

Therefore, to sexually motivate her, you have to really work on making sex so exciting for her so that she considers it a priority.

Attempt Mellow Subjugation And/Or Discipline

For a few ladies, the considered surrendering obligation regarding their sexual fulfillment is an intense turn-on. Set her up by advising her what you will do to her this evening (you can leave her a note or a voice message or send her an email). Request that she get ready for it by wearing your top pick "slave" outfit and making herself lovely. At the point when the time comes, arrange her to get down on her knees and submit to her "expert."

Tie her tenderly with a delicate servitude thing, which can likewise be utilized to gently tease her areolas. You can then continue to tease her with a plume or a tickler, or give her a light punishing with your hand. Sex toys can likewise be utilized here.

Keep in mind: The object of the overwhelming/docile diversion is not mortification or torment; it is to convey her to peak, and conceivably more than once.

Attempt Role Playing

Imagine you are a Penthouse picture taker and welcome her to posture for you, or a pizza conveyance fellow who really likes her, or a policemen capturing her as she is about to escape her auto. This is another variation of investigating her dreams (and yours).

One awesome approach to enjoy what is likely a common dream is to request that her play a stripper or a call young lady with you as her supporter. On the off chance that she appreciates performing for you, you can indeed, even make your own grown-up video and replay it together later on. You would be shocked at what number of ladies fantasize about being in such suggestive parts - just social strictures keep them from letting it be known.

In our general public, which quietly underwrites and advances the Madonna/prostitute dichotomy, giving her consent to showcase her "skanky" dreams or requesting her to "be awful" may very well draw out that skank that you have been longing to have in your room.

Empower Her Sexual Care

Numerous ladies don't get stirred in light of the fact that their brain floats off as opposed to concentrating on the sensuality existing apart from everything else. To direct her musings far from that shopping rundown and to keep her "careful," get her front of the mirror and advise her to watch what you are going to do to her. Verbally depicting every demonstration of foreplay before you do it is additionally a method for keeping her psyche on the warmth existing apart from everything else. Begin by kissing her neck and shoulders as you rub your hands on her dressed body.

At that point, gradually evacuate her underwear yet leave whatever is left of her garments on. Lift her shirt or dress and delicately touch her areolas as you rub her base. Sit her on a seat before the mirror and request her to touch her vulva. You can even request that she rubs some genital warming oil like Zestra on her vaginal lips while you watch. Direct her hands as you inquire her to perform a self-excitement. On the other hand, motivate her to portray her sensations with every move you make. Before long, she will be imploring you to have intercourse with her.

Search her fantasies

Request that her let you know her dreams or to email them to you. Urge her to depict them in point of interest. The closeness that such an admission produces will be sexually stirring for her. Be that as it may, be arranged for the unforeseen. In the event that she reveals that the considered being with another lady (or Brad Pitt) turns her on, don't get bothered or unstable. Rather, misuse it further bolstering your good fortune. While you are kissing and stroking her, turn a storyline that matches her dream. Whisper it in her ear and let her toll in with her own points of interest - which you can use to coordinate your lips and hands. In the event that her psyche likens your touch with her most profound dreams, she will begin getting wet at your first stroke.

Watch Erotica Together

Numerous ladies lean toward aural to visual erotica. Have a go at perusing a hot short story together. Pick one where the "activity" suits your wishes, as well, and read it to her. With regards to visual erotica, numerous ladies lean toward materials that have a plot, and that stress enthusiasm and association between the heroes. That implies leaving your most loved butt-centric bash

DVD for your private autoerotic sessions. Rather, watch a hot adults-only film, for example, 9 1/2 Weeks, or buy an X-appraised video with a storyline by Candida Royalle.

Use Verbal Support

In our general public, which venerates ceaseless youth and frequently sets impossible magnificence models, numerous ladies feel unreliable about their looks and hesitant about their bare bodies. At the point when a lady feels unreliable, she is unrealistic to be in the state of mind for sex. To build her sexual responsiveness, advise her in the middle of kisses and as you touch her body that you locate her excellent and provocative, that she turns you on and that you need to appreciate all aspects of her body before having intercourse to her.

Pay her some particular compliments - advise her you adore her comforting grin, her delicate skin or the shape, size and feel of her bosoms. What's more, don't sit tight for sexual minutes to run out such verbal fortifications.

Be a good Kisser

To be a specialist kisser, begin delicately and work up to more enthusiasm in slow stages. Start by scarcely brushing your lips against hers, and after that touch her lips with the tip of your tongue. Unwind and open your lips as you develop the kiss, yet abstain from dribbling, drooling then again overwhelming vacuum sucking.

On the off chance that you are stressed over terrible breath, make sure to brush your tongue and your teeth, particularly on the off chance that you have been drinking espresso or smoking. In the event that you can't brush, bite on a lemon peel or a mint, or pop a self-dissolving oral consideration strip into your mouth sometime recently starting. You can likewise apply lip medicine with menthol or mint and delicately rub your lips against your accomplice's to share the shiver. Take a stab at keeping eye contact by not shutting your eyes while you kiss. For some ladies, this extends the association and supercharges their sex drive.

Be More Arousing In Your Touches

A greater part of ladies incline toward delicate, delicate touches and strokes everywhere on their body until they get completely stimulated. Sex advisors call this kind of touch "non-interest touch" or "delight centered outer course." Don't simply snatch her bosoms or butt; rather, let your hands gradually achieve those objectives with long, tender touches. When she is completely excited and dribbling with craving, she may love the rougher play, however save that Neanderthal beast in you for the real intercourse.

Lengthen the foreplay

The old cliché is true: Ladies love foreplay. Foreplay does not mean quickly getting her clitoris. Genuine foreplay means beginning as a long way from her private parts as would be prudent - holding her face, stroking her hair, kissing her sanctuaries, looking at her, or rubbing her neck and shoulders. Realize some back rub systems and delicately attempt a couple on her head, neck and shoulders.

Work your direction southward gradually. Take a stab at utilizing only the light touch of your fingertips called pattes d'araignee (the English interpretation "bug legs" some way or another invokes the wrong picture).

Improve the environment

We now and again experience issues blocking boisterously commotions like you're yapping pooch or booming television lights, or disregarding the harmful odors of spoiled nourishment exuding from your untidy kitchen. Yes, that implies killing the TV, darkening the lights, encouraging your pooch, turning up your indoor regulator, taking out the trash and washing the filthy bed covers. In the event that the idea of doing this discourages your sex drive, employ a housekeeper.

Chapter 2: Spicing up your sex life

Learning how to spice up your sex life is something every couple should do. Even if things seem to be going on just well, they can always be better. You can never have enough of your partner. Spicing means trying new stuff or doing things differently. One of the ways to spice our sex life is by learning new sex positions. They always add some freshness and the process of trying them out is so much fun. In the second section of this book, we shall exclusively look at some sex positions couples should try out.

Sexual fetishes

Fetishes are using body parts, objects or materials to lead up to an elevated state of sexual arousal. They may also be referred to as sexual preferences or kinks. These enhance the sexual experiences in a manner that normal sex wouldn't. For couples, it can be a good way to improve your sex life. Talking about sexual fetishes with your partner and actually trying them out can lead to deep sexual satisfaction. The key here is to talk about it as some fetishes might cross your partner's boundaries. However, if it does no harm, doesn't compromise one's beliefs and is legal, then there shouldn't be a reason not to try it out. Keep in mind that the fetish doesn't have to be performed each time you indulge in sex rather occasionally to heighten the pleasure. In fact, a fetish doesn't always need to be performed; even talking about it can bring so much pleasure to some people. Exploring each other fetishes means you are both very comfortable with other and intimately close. You can initiate the conversation with your partner regarding anything special that they'd like to try out in the bedroom.

Talking dirty to your partner

Is there anybody who doesn't love some dirty talk from their partner? I doubt there is. Dirty talk is one way in which couples can bring back the oomph to their sex life. Couples should seize every opportunity available to tell each other how much they want them and what they need them to do. Even if the situation doesn't allow you to jump into each other's arms, you'll slowly build the anticipation and by the time you hit the sack, everything will just be waiting to explode. When having sex, always talk with your partner and let them know how they make you feel. Men, in particular, are turned on by dirty talking during sex. Women, on the other hand, love dirty talk before sex to bring them to the mood. You can send each other sexy sex messages during the day. You don't have to be very creative with words. Just a simple phrase lets your partner knows you are thinking about them and you can't wait to have them.

It might seem awkward to initiate dirty talk if you haven't been doing it before but it's worth it. Just try it maybe at first using a text message before you say it to your partner. These small things make all the difference.

Rekindling romance

After the initial excitement fizzles out, it is possible to get into a rut. Rekindling romance improves our sex life as well. Romance and sex go hand in hand. However, we shouldn't confuse sex for romance, like most men are likely to do. But when a partner feels loved and appreciated, they open up more leading to better sex. Without romance, our sex lives are the first to suffer. We might find ourselves just going through the motions without really achieving much emotionally. Romance can be rekindled by expressing your desire for your partner and appreciating them. Go out for dates every once in a while and always make an effort to please your partner. If you have kids, take some time when you can have someone look after them and just enjoy each other's company with no distractions at all. Plan for a honeymoon vacation every year to reconnect with your partner is another option. Our professional lives can eat up so much of our time that we lose the connection with our partner. Talk with your partner daily not just about the kids or the finances but also about yourselves. This makes you know your partner more and understand them. Believe me, even people married for decades have something new to learn about their partner. Engaging in a new activity can help you spend more time together. You might pick a new hobby, pick an exercise plan or just make a point of going out more often. All these will translate to a better sex life due to the increased intimacy and connection.

Spontaneous vs. scheduled sex

We plan everything important in life be it meetings, doctor's appointments, meeting with friends and anything else in between. But when it comes to sex, most of us cringe at the idea of scheduling sex. Spontaneous sex is the best, everybody agrees, but our busy schedules often don't allow time for it. People are working more and more hours. Partners can often feel like roommates when their schedules crash or one of them is too tired or not in the mood. This is where setting aside time for sex can really play an important role. At this time, sex is the number one priority, it's the only thing. Everything else is set aside and we focus on making love. Younger lovers might find this idea not quite appealing but it can help if you find yourselves having no time for sex. However, scheduling sex doesn't mean you can't have the spontaneous sex when possible. In fact you should also plan for spontaneity. This is by having in place anything you require for sex at the right place for when you have sex. If you use condoms or lubricants, realizing just before you have sex that you don't have any left can be quite a disappointment.

Chapter 3: Sexual Self-esteem

Insecurity is one of the critical factors that limit people's sexual life. In my teenage years and early youth, I was way insecure. To top it up even further, I was also a premature ejaculator, except for a magical and premonitory encounter at the age of 14 that introduced me intuitively to the alchemy of the integrated enjoyment of body, heart, and consciousness. I was blessed by a spontaneous orgasmic encounter, desired by both of us who placed us in the middle of the forest looking at the stars together, hallucinated by a sense of timeless magic. That experience was a key reference to transcend the normal sexuality of anxious men.

My self-esteem difficulties were overcome with an intense and committed interior work and with the contributions of loving beings, who provided signs of light and affection. Thus, I learned to value myself as a person and a man, affirming my condition as an intensely masculine non-macho man, without denying my sensitivity and joy of experiencing sexual enjoyment in harmony with a loving and non-sinful conscience.

The worst problems of human sexuality are verified around insecurity. Many of the roads to perversion start from there. This book is not just preventive, but it also promotes the good character of full sexuality. It will definitely not deepen the negative aspects associated with the difficulties of sexual self-esteem. I prefer to highlight the possibilities of internalizing positive sexual self-esteem.

In my life, the improvement of my personal esteem coincided with access to fuller sexuality. Since then, a feeling of inner security blesses me. It enhances my sexual capacity, enabling me to share pleasure and love. It helps me experiencing the conscious joy of being alive, traveling and being in a universe along with my partner.

It is difficult for a woman to have positive sexual self-esteem. Phrases like "to be good for sex" or to notice that "she likes sex" have meant the condemnation of these valuable women. They are wrongly labeled as seemingly serious, not fit for the role of holy mothers and selfless wives. In the case of men, exhibitionist machismo has cultivated different images to prove sexual superpowers: penis size, resistance in time, amount of intercourse in a meeting, the number of women conquered, etc.

Beyond these complications and categories, feeling sexually attractive and trained to cause loving pleasure in your partner is a great feeling that cooperates with the integral development of people. Learning and practicing a more evolved sexuality is a vital sign of growth and self-realization. The dense and negative burden of low sexual self-esteem is absolutely overcome with inner discipline, empathy, and kindness in establishing relationships with others.

The Energy of Sex

A century ago, Albert Einstein translated the existence of energy into scientific certainty.

Current science recognizes that all the bodies of the universe are a dynamic matter-energy conversion, materially and energetically connected with other bodies, all integrated into ecosystems to which we belong.

To be honest, we are the energy interacting with the void and the different levels of matter. The impulses of our nervous networks act sequentially as energetic waves and material corpuscles.

Our beings and bodies vibrate with energy. It is essential to recognize it, integrate it, and use it harmoniously for our benefit.

The current way of life (focused on the matter) has little expertise in the harmonic control of our energy flows. In their ignorance, the "normal people" have given the character of "esoteric" to the practices of human energy development. Therefore, from the traditional point of view, those who participate in these experiences appear strange and suspicious.

The poor sexual education that most people receive is conceived from a limited perspective that mixes a materialistic view of the human body, with a traditional moralizing discourse. The body is a lot of "parts" and the moral and spirit appear dissociated from it. For the purposes of this work, we will understand the human body as a physiological and energetic unit, that is, a functioning body - system, animated by multidimensional energy flows.

What happens during sexual encounters is an intense exchange of matter and energy, producing powerful transformations of all kinds in our integral being. A

22

wonderful world of stimuli to recognize a millenary and updated principle of wisdom:

"We are part of a bustling universe of energy which is in permanent transformation, moving towards the indeterminate."

The illusion of a "static and predictable security" at the service of the human being trembles before the coincident visions of quantum physics, ancestral wisdom, astronomy, and ecological understanding of our place in the cosmos. We are definitely not the center of the universe and it does not revolve around us. In a universe still of undetermined limits, it is an illusory game to seek its center, madness to believe that we are that center. We flow in an ocean of changing life. We are a mobile, interactive part with millions of possible combinations of encounters.

Medicine and the scientific study of the human being in the west slowly begin to integrate the other side of body reality: "energy". Acupuncture and other alternative health practices are now accepted as auxiliary techniques of Public and Private Health (Old knowledge about meridians and energy flows is already assumed).

Just as water, blood, and liquids of different compositions flow through our material body (constituting almost 80% of our total matter), we are also covered by energy flows. Energy training has been key in my sexual self-realization. I think that basically, love is made, sex is shared from "energy", and energy is what is radiated from genital and bodily sensations, feelings, and perceptions of conscience.

To improve personal sex life, it is crucial to achieve the development of the energetic perception of reality and the ability to use the flow of energy that each one possesses dynamically and harmoniously. I recommend readers to be open to learning the functional and energetic reality of our bodies. I suggest you use the passion of a researcher in the sensitive and specific perception of the bodies – the energies of our partners.

Sexual love with its wise mixture of subtlety and intensity effectively links the material body with the spiritual one. It is a unitary process which is full of life and has the potential for harmony.

In the second and third part of this book, we will see that the control and transmutation techniques of seminal ejaculation are based on energy training. The warning signal of ejaculation is the first impulse of energy. The woman in her orgasmic peaks lives an "experience of energy expansion" accompanied by lubricating and hormonal flows.

In order to perform the exercises recommended in the second part of this book, it is necessary for the reader to practice the energy training exercises included in the third part of this book, especially the ones dedicated to "recognition, integration, and balance of energetic flows and chakras of the human being".

It is necessary, before starting to work with internal energy, to specify the meaning of the word "chakra". "Chakra" is usually translated as "energy center", which leads to the error of locating them as a "material place" in some physical area of the body.

In Sanskrit, "chakra" means wheel, which reinforces the understanding of energy as movement and multidirectional flow. In this book, we will understand chakra: those spaces - times of energy confluence referenced in certain areas of the body in which the basic energy that the human being shares with the universe is specified in certain levels of functioning.

The specific location in an area of the body will facilitate the "energy - spatial perception" of the chakra. Breathing and, in other cases, visualization will be the techniques and instruments that will facilitate access to a "spiritual experience of our being". The proposed exercises are key experiences for the development of good sex. Its practice has meant for me: a constant renewal of my energy flow, obtaining valuable information about my real inner state, and the discovery of expedited channels to harmonize and transform my sexual energy.

Chapter 4: 17 Sexual and Aphrodisiacs Food

Eating the right food is not just vital for your overall health; it can also help you to achieve much better performance in the bedroom department. You must eat foods that are full of the nutrients you need to promote good sexual health. Those nutrients are:

- Amino acids
- Niacin
- Phosphorus
- Potassium
- Vitamin-B complex
- Vitamin B6
- Vitamin B12
- Zinc

Provided you are feeding your body all of these vital nutrients, plus other vitamins and minerals, you can be sure that your performance will significantly improve over time and you can knock premature ejaculation on the head.

Poor diets are responsible for a lot of things, not least poor sexual performance, low levels of testosterone, a low quality of erection, no sex drive, impotence, no libido and premature ejaculation. Eating a good diet will clear up all of that and more, as well as helping you to last much longer in bed.

Think about that before you start popping pills and sing creams and sprays; sometimes all you need to do is change the way you eat.

So, what are these performance-boosting foods then?

Leafy Green Vegetables

Eat plenty of these on a daily basis to increase your performance and improve your sexual health. Make sure you eat a good selection, including:

- Collards
- Kale
- Spinach
- Swiss chard
- Beet greens

Oatmeal

Oatmeal is a true power food, especially when it comes to sex. Eating oatmeal on a regular basis will provide you with a significant increase in energy levels and a boost in performance, helping you to stay the pace for a lot longer

Cereals

Eating a bowl of cereal at breakfast time will provide you with a range of the important nutrients you need. It will also help you to store energy for longer, resulting in a much better performance in bed

Nuts

Nuts should be a daily part of your diet to keep you healthy, active and energetic:

- Almonds
- Brazil nuts
- Butternuts
- Hazelnut
- Hickory nut
- Peanuts
- Pine nuts
- Pistachio
- Walnuts

All of these are packed full of powerful antioxidants and sex nutrients

Whole Grain

This is another fantastic food for helping to improve your stamina and improve your performance

Sunflower Seeds

These are perhaps the best of all the seeds, a real power food. Enjoy them on their own, on a salad, over a fish and vegetable meal, or you can blend them up in a sauce or a soup

Celery

Celery is a true powerhouse and you can eat it in a number of ways. Raw, add it to a salad or juice it with cucumber, spinach and lemon for a sexy smoothie. Try to drink one liter a day to really improve things in bed

Liver

Lamb and beef liver are full of B-vitamins and are extremely important for men and sex. They can help to increase your sperm count, your sexual desire, and your libido, as well as improving your performance

Steak

Steak contains a high level of sex nutrients making it one of the best foods to eat. It also raises the dopamine levels in your bloodstream, helping you to be more aware of when you are about to ejaculate, giving you time to hold it back and get it under control

Salmon

Salmon is another good food for building up sexual stamina. They are full of nutrients and omega 3 fatty acid, providing you with everything you need for a top performance between the sheets

Oysters

The original aphrodisiac, the humble oyster is a true superhero for improving sexual health

Lobster

Lobster has long been linked to a healthy and strong male libido and is packed full of nutrients that can help to boost your sex drive and increase your sensitivity towards sex

Honey

Honey provides you with energy that will keep you on the go all night. Just add a spoonful or two of honey to a glass of milk and eat a handful of nuts before bed to give you plenty of energy and help you to last a lot longer in bed.

Dark Chocolate

Chocolate is actually good for you, provided you eat dark chocolate with a high cocoa content. It provides a boost to your energy levels but do watch how much you eat – it will quickly add calories to your diet

Yogurt

Eating a cup of yogurt, nonfat variety, with a few blueberries provides you with one of the best sex foods of all time. Add a little of that honey to it and you will be raring to go – and keep on going. Try eating a yogurt for breakfast, mixed with nuts and seeds as well

Ice Cream

Especially the good old vanilla flavor can increase your sex drive quite significantly. If you like to experiment with food during sex, you can't go wrong with vanilla ice cream. Not only will the smell work to relax you, your inhibitions will be lowered and you will have a much longer-lasting power to keep going

Bananas

Eating bananas on a regular basis will give your sex life a real boost and provide you with lasting energy. They are packed full of potassium and Vitamin-B complex which are two of the most powerful of all the sex nutrients.

They won't stop you from having a premature ejaculation but they will give you the power to keep ongoing.

NOTE – Make sure you eat raw foods where you can and stick to organic. These contain the most nutrients, minerals and vitamins and have much less in the way of harmful chemicals.

So, there you go, 17 foods that are guaranteed to boost your sex life, increase your sex drive and help you to last longer in bed. Add in regular exercise and you will soon be seeing some fantastic change and sexual benefits

Chapter 5: 5 Shocking Things That Can Help You Last Longer in Bed

If there are two things that most men are insecure about, whether they admit it or not, it is sex and the size of their penis. All men, no matter what walk of life they come from, like to be proud of the size of their lunchbox and of how long they can last in bed, simply because they are of the belief that a bigger than average size and the ability to last much longer are the two things that build up the sexual appetite of the woman they are with. Unfortunately, there is little they can do about the size of their tools, they can do something to make themselves last a god deal longer in bed.

While it can be an advantage in some things to be able to finish quickly, sex is not one of them. In fact, premature ejaculation is one of the most common of all the sexual problems that a man suffers from and is also the most distressing for both parties. Recent research found that an immense 45% of men finish too quickly, within two minutes of starting sex. The average time for sex is 7.3 minutes, about 4 minutes less than the average woman would like it to last.

OK, so this is probably quite discouraging for both men and women but it is important to remember that both stamina and performance can be enhanced and improved in some unlikely ways. Here are just five of those ways:

1. A big belly

Contrary to what you have been told, size really does matter in terms of sex. Unfortunately, it isn't the size of your tool, it is the size of your belly. A study published in 2010 in The Journal of Sexual Medicine, said that men with bigger bellies made better lovers. Men, who were overweight, with an obviously larger belly, were lasting the average of 7.3 minutes while thinner men could hardly make it to the two-minute mark. This might seem to be somewhat counterintuitive but, the researchers determined that the more belly fat a man has, the higher the level of estradiol, which is the female sex hormone, and this is what helps to slow the orgasm down.

2. Adult Circumcision

We've all heard the phrase, "better late than never", and we all know that it can apply in a number of different ways, and that includes adult circumcision. In 204, a study that was published in the Adult Urology journal revealed that men who were circumcised took quite a bit longer to ejaculate, after being circumcised as an adult. While some people will believe this to be a hindrance, there are those, particularly those who suffer from premature ejaculation, who will see this as a blessing. The study originated in the GATA Haydarpasa Training Hospital in Istanbul and was carried out by urologist Temucin Senkul. He determined that the delay was down to the circumcision having an effect on penis sensitivity

3. Exercise – Pelvic Floor

These exercises are not just for women or for people who have problems with their bladder; they can also be of great help in treating premature ejaculation. The European Congress of Urology in Stockholm carried out a study on 40 men, aged between 19 and 46, who averaged 31.7 seconds for ejaculation. They were set 12 weeks of pelvic floor exercises and, at the end, 33 of the men showed a marked improvement in ejaculation time along with a significant increase in self-confidence. By the end of the 12 weeks, the average time had risen to 146.2 seconds, almost four times what it was at the start of the research.

4. A Vegetarian Diet

If there is one thing that staunch vegetarians are known for, it is the strength of the stance they take on dairy and meat intake. However, they are also known for being able to last longer in bed, because of an increase in both energy and stamina. Vegan diets, high in fruit, can give you a much higher level of sustainable energy, that will not be subject to the "sugar crash" that we often see with a typical western diet packed full of processed sugars. Bananas, for example, are very high in potassium, which is a nutrient helpful to the production of sex hormones and for boosting energy levels.

Various and numerous tests have shown that those who eat a vegetarian diet have got twice the level of stamina than a meat-eater. The Yale Medical Journal published a study that compared athletes who ate meat to athletes who were vegetarian or near-vegetarian – half of these latter groups led a sedentary lifestyle. The research involved measuring how long each person in the study could hold their arms outstretched and how many deep knee bends they could do. Just 13% of the meat-eaters could keep their arms outstretched for 15 minutes, compared to a whopping 69% of vegetarians. None of the meat-eaters could keep their arms out for 30 minutes while 4% of the vegetarians could. With the knee bends, 33% of meat-eaters managed more than 352, against 81% of the vegetarians.

5. Viagra

The famous little blue pill. While it was mainly used to treat impotence or erectile dysfunction, it also has its uses when it comes to giving the sexual performance a boost. The magic ingredients in Viagra are phosphodiesterase-5 inhibitors, female hormones that delay orgasm. A 2012 study that was published in the Journal of Sexual Medicine showed that the pill could help men to extend the lime they lasted in bed before they had an orgasm.

Out of 14 studies, 11 of them showed that the medication could be associated with lasting longer in bed but not all of the studies could say for definite if Viagra was the responsible ingredient as it was never tested against anything else, most specifically a placebo.

When it comes to premature ejaculation, the key to beating it, or to improve your sexual stamina, can be down to something as simple as mind over matter. Athletes have to practice hard to increase their stamina and their energy levels and the same is true of sex. At the end of the day, there isn't a problem that can't be got over so get practicing.

Chapter 6: Different Types of Sexual Play

There are many different types of sex. There's role-playing, public, naughty, kinky, domination, and so on. And while some of them may seem downright odd to you or your partner, I would suggest trying a mild version of all of these in order to figure out what you two like in the bedroom together. Half the battle of having a great sex life knows what your partner likes, and the other half knows what you like. So educate yourself on the different techniques in this chapter!

Role-playing

Everyone has fantasies, and if you're involved in a dedicated relationship and you think about a hot police officer with some cuffs, don't be shy about asking your significant other to play out that fantasy. Role-playing is a thrill for both people involved, and it gives partners that thrill of sleeping with other people without actually sleeping with others. It's a really great way to keep monogamy really hot. If you don't know where to begin with this type of sex, try the class 'we don't know each other' sex. It gives you both the freedom to act as if you're someone else and take on a different personality, and allows you to do things you've always wanted to do but were afraid to ask to do.

Exercise: Try going out to a restaurant with a bar attached and wait for your significant other to show up. Have them know what is happening and pretend that the two of you don't know each other. You can also do this if you go to a park if you want it to be a little more secluded and private.

Splurge Sex

Have you ever noticed that when you go to a really nice place with your partner, the two of you seem to be amped up? Well, this is a phenomenon that occurs because the two of you are really excited about where you're at because it's different. So when you book that next vacation, splurge and go for a really nice room for at least one night so that the two of you can have a relaxing, adventurous day. You can even rent a hotel room in a city or town nearby that you know is really nice for one night, even if you're not going on vacation.

Public Sex

I'm not suggesting you get it on in the bathroom of a club, but if that's your thing, go for it. I am suggesting that if you go to the movies sit in the back row and guide his or her hand somewhere that's a little naughty. You don't have to do the entire deed in public, but get it started a little before you drive home to have some of the best sex of your life!

Beach Sex

There is a drink named after this act of sex on the beach, so it has to amazing, right? You'll enjoy the crashing waves, the sun, and your hot partner with you. You don't have to limit yourself to lying down in the sand. The two of you could take a beach blanket, a lounge chair, or even have sex in the water.

Forbidden Sex

There's a book all about forbidden sex, and it's been a best seller for quite some time. Women and men both enjoy a little bit of kinkiness in the bedroom, so get out those handcuffs and figure out who's going to be the dominant one and who will be the submissive one for the evening. You don't have to live the BDSM lifestyle in order to try out a little taste of it.

Bathroom Sex

This is the most underrated room in the entire house for having sex. Seriously, it's a really great room! Try bending over the counter in doggie style position as your partner is behind you and watches his face as he takes you. Or sit on the counter so that he can see your backside at the same time that he's fondling your front. Men like a woman's sexy back and seeing the flow of her hair down her shoulders.

Makeup Sex

There are plenty of couples out there who will start a fight just because they know they're going to get makeup sex. I'm not kidding! Make up sex is charged with all that emotion that you just experienced, and it can be really steamy and hot. Women, don't resist the urge to have sex with a man after a fight. You're punishing yourself just as much as you're punishing him.

Lazy Sex

Sex does not have to be a marathon or a crazy ten-minute bout in the bedroom. The next time you're feeling lazy in the afternoon or it's the morning and the weekend, take off all your clothes and snuggle up to your partner. Men and women's hormone levels are higher in the morning and early afternoon, so it's a great time to have some really slow, connecting sex.

Loud Sex

All those four-letter words that you would never say in polite company are the ones that you want to use in the bedroom at least once during your relationship. Seriously, go all out and tell your partner exactly what you want him or her to do to you. Let them know how much you like it. The more explicit you are and the louder you are, the more excited they're guaranteed to be.

Random Sex

You know those times when you least expect your partner to jump your bones, and it happened? They were pretty exciting times, right? Well, return the favor to them! The next time you're walking through a secluded park and it seems there isn't anyone else around, pull your partner to a private spot and get it on!

Chapter 7: Playing in Public

That feeling of doing something dirty at the risk of getting caught can be such a turn on and build a bond between you and your partner. The delayed gratification of slow foreplay and the build-up to hot and heavy sex is something that every couple should experience together.

Sex at Dinner

Go to a nice restaurant. One where you should be on your best, if not decent, behavior. Start with a couple of dirty texts at the table, maybe some footie under the table. Text each other what you want to do in that moment and watch your partner squirm with excitement.

At some point in the night, both of you will take a turn going to the bathroom and sending a naughty photo to the other, which must be opened discretely at the table. Fuck each other with your eyes and then when you get back to the car, take a few minutes to release some of that sexual tension.

At the Movie Theatre

It's dark, it's loud and it's the perfect place to do everything and anything to each other's' bodies. Hand jobs and fingering are an easy escapade to accomplish in a crowded theatre. She can reach over for a little tug action, and she can lay her legs across her man's lap giving him full access. If you are more daring than 2nd base, you'd better sit in the back.

The back row is the perfect place for a sneaky blowjob or even full penetration as she sits on his lap.

Pro Tip: Go to a movie that's been out for weeks and you're more likely to get a bit of privacy.

Remote Control Bullet Vibrator

Vibrator bullets fit perfectly up her pussy, while her partner holds the remote control. He can increase the vibrators' speed and change up the settings whenever and where he likes.

Before dinner, slip the vibrator in her pussy and tell her that you're going to have a little fun. The vibrator is small enough that she may even forget that it's inside of her...at least until he turns it on while the waiter is taking her order.

Finger Her in the Car

To get ready for this naughty play, wear a skirt or a dress; something with easy access. Start by rubbing and then slide a few fingers in when she's really wet.

Pro Tip: If you don't have tinted windows, you'll have to be sneaky about this one.

Road Head

Driving on the back roads or driving at night is the perfect time to unzip his pants and have a little fun on the drive home. Make sure he keeps his eyes on the road, otherwise he may have to pull over if he gets really into it.

Sex on the Top of a Mountain

Yes, really. Go on a hike together. Get those endorphins pumping and get a little sweaty. Find a remote spot (preferably with a view) and bend her over a tree or find some soft grass to lay down in. Just make sure that you are totally isolated...which theoretically, shouldn't be too difficult.

Camping Sex

Whether you pitch a literal and figurative tent in the back yard or in the wilderness, the change of scenery is titillating. It will either be just the two of you having loud passionate sex with the acoustics of the forest or you'll have to muffle her screams so that your camping neighbors don't hear your real-life porno.

Sex in a Public Restroom

Scope out your spot. As you go out to eat or meet for drinks, be on the lookout for bathrooms that will grant you enough privacy to get it on. Then...pick a night for the fun to begin.

She'll get up first to use the restroom. He'll follow quickly behind. She'll already have her panties slid to the side while she's playing with herself and ready for him to enter her. He may have to cover her mouth while he bends her over, just to be discrete.

Pro Tip: Have hot bathroom sex after you've paid your bill. Your waiter won't be looking for you and you can make a sneaky exit once you've finished.

Visit a Swingers Club

Sex Club, Swingers Club, Kink Club...whatever you can find in your area – every city has one!

If you've never been to a sex club before, the thought alone can be terrifying. But there is a role for everyone's comfort zone here. Which role do you fit into?

Curious Folk: People who are new to the concept of sex clubs and just want to check it out.

Voyeurs: Those who just like to watch.

Exhibitionists: People who like to have sex in front of other people.

Swingers: Couples that like to swap and share partners with other couples.

Everyone is welcome in a sex club! No one will push you guys to do anything you don't want to do. You won't be pressured to get involved. And you won't be the only first-timers there!

This is the kind of night where you and your partner will really lean on each other in a foreign environment. You'll have that adrenaline pumping and endorphins flowing, all while you're next to each other doing something that feels so...taboo.

Chapter 8: Experimental Sexual Positions

You may not have tried tantric sex, but perhaps it's time you did. The idea of Tantric sex goes back generations and the Kama Sutra explained all about it. This was a book written by a priest and the intention of the book was to allow couples to find perfect harmony in their marriages, so that the love lasted longer and the couple found close bonding within their relationship. The same applies today and you can experiment with different lovemaking techniques that enhance your love life. She will love you for it because all of these practices are caring and that's the nature of a woman.

When you decide to try Tantric sex, you will need to have warmed coconut oil for massage that leads to lovemaking. You will also need to prepare the bedroom so that it is a temple of pleasure. Make sure that you protect your sheets with large towels and that you have both discussed tantric sex in advance. Choose an evening when you have lots of time on your hands and you know you won't be interrupted.

Massage plays a large role in the kind of sexual activity you share with your partner. It's all about satisfying your partner, rather than yourself. Massaging her clitoris isn't all there is to it. Massage inside her and find her G spot. Massage the area of the anus as well if you have both consented to it. You will find that this area actually links with her G spot internally and that you are likely to get a very marked response to this massage. Similarly, she can massage you and the most sensitive area she can massage is the area between the testicles and the back passage because it is here that all of your sexual senses are awakened.

Positions suitable to tantric sex

Closeness and intimacy is everything when you are making love in the tantric way. You may decide that you want to pleasure her in a gentle way and letting her sit on your lap and then sitting up to join her is a good way to start making love. Your bodies will slide together and she will be able to hold onto you or lean back so that you can play with her clitoris as well as entering her vagina. Again, slow rocking will help you to excite each other and you need to learn to hold off on climaxing. When you feel she is near climax, stop. Then start all over again. The idea of tantric sex is to make the climax something explosive and the more you hold off on climaxing the huger the climax will become. Make sure that you are both on the same page. You can read the Kama Sutra together and try many of the intimate positions suggested, making sure that the climax isn't the whole focus of lovemaking. The focus is on improving the pleasure for your partner and extending that pleasure.

The Bow – This position is a very powerful position and allows full penetration. It also allows a man maximum thrust while a woman's hands can be used to massage the testicles. The woman lies on her back and places her feet onto the chest of her man who is kneeling between her legs. Her behind is raised and you may find it more comfortable if you use a cushion so that the level is perfect for entry into her. Before entering her, make sure that she is massaged and that the oils allow easy penetration. Get her to push against your chest with her feet because this gives you more thrust and more control over the lovemaking process. While you are making love in this way, she can massage you and this helps to make your orgasm even stronger.

Crossed leg lovemaking – This may sound like a contradiction in terms, but it is the position that derives this title because of the stance taken. A man lays his woman onto a table edge. Her legs are lifted to his shoulders but before placing them onto his shoulders, he crosses her legs. You may wonder why the crossing of the legs is so essential but this is because of the woman's anatomy. It gives her greater control over the muscles within the vagina and she is able to move her body in rhythm with his so that she gains maximum thrust and he gains maximum friction. It's a wonderful way to make love and something that will make both the man and the woman very happy indeed.

If you introduce tantric sexual practices into your lovemaking, you will find that you will be less shy of each other and will be able to share a lot more of your desires with your partner as well as being open to listen to hers. She may have a wealth of ideas that will spice up your love life, but she needs to have total trust in your reactions. Be open and talk to her. Let her know that the rules of the bedroom are that she can feel free to talk about her own sexual desires as well as fulfilling yours. Many women are a little shy about talking about sex, so will need that level of reassurance that helps them to open up and be honest. It isn't lack of honesty. It's being afraid of your reactions that make a woman hold back from being adventurous. Show her that you want her to be happy in bed and listen to what she says. She may have ideas that will fill your lovemaking with a new sense of happiness and contentment.

Chapter 9: Sex Positions for Beginners

If you are a novice when it comes to sex, the act can seem really intimidating and overwhelming. When you enter into a sexual relationship, it takes time for you to learn what you like, what your partner likes, and what balance strikes the best chord with you both. Getting tense and worrying about the situation only makes it worse, so my first piece of advice is to take a deep breath and allow yourself to relax. Allow things to move at a natural pace and do not try to rush. Start off with simple positions that are not too challenging so that you can focus on the feelings they arouse. This will allow you to feel connected and safe with your partner. Here are a few simple sex positions that every beginner should try.

Missionary Position

This position is famous for its simplicity and the great variation that it allows for both partners. By simply changing the angle of your legs, you can change the sensations aroused from this position. It allows for a deep feeling of connection between partners while allowing deep penetration. It is also one of the most common positions that allow women to orgasm from penetrative sex. This is due to the fact that the man's penis is more likely to hit the woman's g-spot with inward strokes of his penis. To get started with the basic missionary position, the woman lies on her back and the man gets into position between her spread thighs so that their pubic regions are aligned and penetration is possible.

Lying Face to Face

This position is great for beginners as it allows you to both be comfortable and be in tune with each other's needs because of the intimacy it creates due to the eye contact and deep penetration. To do this position, all you have to do is lie on your sides facing each other. The woman should lie slightly higher than the man with her hips above his. She should then place her top leg over his hips and allow his penis to slide inside of her.

Spooning

This position is great for G-spot stimulation and allows for lots of skin-to-skin contact. It is like cuddling and sex in one. The man can easily reach around and stimulate the woman's clit in this position. This is a simple position for couples to achieve. Lay in a spooning position with the woman's hips slightly above the man's. Her top leg should be slightly lifted so that he can penetrate her.

Woman on Top

In this position, the woman straddles the man while he sits so that their faces are close together. This position allows the woman more control but still allows the couple to be connected emotionally. To get in this position, the man must be seated and reclined against something like a couch or a wall. The woman straddles him until their genitals are aligned and penetration is possible.

Doggy Style

This position is great for deeper penetration and leaves both the man's and woman's hands-free for clitoral play and stimulation. To get into this position, the woman rests on her hands and knees with her legs spread so that her partner can get behind her. She can adjust the width of her legs closer or wider to accommodate height differences and to allow for the variations in penetration.

Experimental Sexual Positions for Beginners

Variety is the spice of life, and this is also true for sex. Doing the same positions over and over again can quickly become boring and make a couple's sex life become stagnant. This does not have to happen to you and your partner. Even if you are both beginners to sex, you can switch things up and keep things spicy with the position outlined below.

Missionary Position Variations

Remember that I said that the missionary position allows for great versatility. By lifting the woman's feet off the bed and pushing her knees closer to her chest, this variation in the missionary position allows for deeper penetration and greater access to the G-spot. If the woman is particularly limber, she can place her ankles on the man's shoulders for an even greater lift of her buttocks off the surface that they are lying on.

You can also alter the missionary position by placing a pillow underneath the woman's hips. This missionary variation allows the man's body to rub against the woman's clitoris with every inward stroke of his penis. This makes the woman more likely to orgasm from the position.

In the missionary position, you can also experiment with the woman lifting one leg at a time and having the man lift his chest at different angles away from her body. Small things can make a huge difference, and the variations that you can add to the missionary position are a testament to that fact.

Modified Doggy Style

This position is great for participating in dirty talk as the man's mouth is close to the woman's ear. In this position, the woman lies on her stomach with her hips tilted towards the man who lies behind her. A pillow under the woman's hips can allow the couple to find the right angle for pleasurable penetration. In addition, this is a great position for a woman who would like to show off her derriere to her partner if it is a feature that she is proud of.

Dangling Over the Bed

This position is easy on a man's body as it does not require him to hold his body up with his arms. Since the woman is lying on the edge of a bed with her legs hanging off, he simply has to place himself between her thighs, penetrate her, and thrust them both to a happy finish.

Sex Positions to Help You Get Over Insecurities

Having body issues and feeling insecure about your body is not something that is new, and both men and women suffer from the condition that can sometimes be debilitating. These insecurities can, of course, transfer into your sex life as you need to bare your body to have good sex. The great thing about having a supportive sex partner is that they can help you get over these insecurities and perceived flaws since most of the time we are a lot harder on ourselves and see flaws that other people do not.

Of course, you can help get over these insecurities by addressing them in individual ways such as going to the gym and dieting if you feel that you are overweight. In the bedroom, to help get over your insecurities, a great technique is to find the positions that highlight the features you find most attractive about yourself.

Before we look at some of the sex positions that will allow you to feel less insecure about your body, there are a few other things that you can do to boost your self-confidence in your physical appearance:

- **Learn to love yourself and build your self-esteem.** No matter the sexual positions that you try, if, at the end of the day, you do not love yourself for who you are and what you look like, your insecurities will always rear their head.

- **Spend more time naked.** Get familiar with what it feels like to be naked and become intimate with your own body so that when it comes time to be sexually intimate with your partner, you are less likely to be uncomfortable in your own skin.

- **Disassociate with people who speak negatively to you about you.** Associating with toxic people who not only talk negatively about your body but about their own has a negative impact on you. Therefore, if you have people like this in your life, it is time to have a frank and open discussion about how their words affect you, and if they are not willing to change, then you need to think about cutting them out of your life.

Without further ado, here are a few sexual positions that will encourage you to have a better body image about yourself:

Cowgirl

This position is great for helping you get over insecurities because it brings any issues that may be had to the forefront so that they can be dealt with. For example, if a woman is insecure about her breasts, in this position her partner has a full view of them and can reassure her of her beauty and uniqueness. This is also a great position for a woman who feels that her breasts are one of her best assets and wants to show them off to her partner.

This position is great for beginners because it provides body views and great eye contact. To get into this position, the woman straddles her partner and guides his penis to penetrate her. She should use her hands and knees for balance. She bounces her hips up and down to provide stimulation to both herself and her partner. The man can aid this by lifting his hips up and down as well and supporting her with his arms. In this position, the woman can control the speed and intensity of the strokes. She can also widen her knees or bring them closer to change the depth of penetration.

The Three-Legged Dog Position

This position is great for the promotion of dirty talk and having eye contact in addition to having full upper body contact. It allows both partners to concentrate on their emotional connection rather than physical appearances. Therefore, it is great for people with insecurities since the emphasis is placed on eye contact rather than on each other's bodies. This position involves both parties standing. To aid with equilibrium, one party can lean against a wall. The woman leans into the man with her legs separated and hikes one leg over his hips so that he can penetrate her.

In a Chair

This position is great for reassuring insecurities for the same reasons that the above position is. It allows for lots of upper body contact and lots of eye contact. In this position, the man sits in a chair and the woman straddles him with her thighs on either side of his body. She can bounce up and down or grind against him to stimulate them both.

Lotus

In this position, the man sits crossed-legged on a flat, comfortable surface, and the woman sits on his lap so that they are facing each other. She wraps her legs and arms around him. They can both aid in the penetration and stimulation of each other. This position helps both parties feel secure in the fact that they are emotionally connected with eye contact. Just like the spooning position, this is sex and cuddling in one, and all the associated feel-good hormones are released when couples engage in sex in this position.

Chapter 10: Quick and Easy When you just have time for a quickie.

Sometimes you don't have the time, energy or inclination to have a long sex session, it may even be inappropriate to do so. Quickie sex can be every bit as satisfying as longer sex sessions because there is a lot less pressure – you know that you both want to do your thing and get it over with.

Quickies are also ideal for adding a special element of excitement when it comes to sex. Maybe you and your partner can have a quickie in the powder room at the next wedding you go to, or maybe add a frisson of excitement by doing over the hood of the car. Many people have a fantasy of having sex in a public place and this is the ideal time to have a quickie.

Take your quickies up to the next level by using the advanced sex positions in this book. These positions do require a bit of effort but are deeply satisfying and give intense pleasure. They are designed for quick stimulation and are not maintainable for too long unless you are both very athletic.

Raised Doggy Style

Your hum-drum doggie style can be taken up a notch if done in a standing position. The woman starts by bending over and placing her hands flat on the floor, facing away from the man. The man lifts the woman up by the hips and penetrates while she extends her legs straight out behind her. This makes for an interesting variation but does require that the man is fairly fit.

The Side Saddle

The man sits on the edge of a bed or a chair without arms, legs together. The woman lowers herself onto his lap, facing to the side of him at a ninety-degree angle. This can be a challenging pose for the woman.

The Lift-Off

The two of you need to stand face to face. The man must then pick the woman up and penetrate her while she wraps her legs around his waist. If need be, this can be done up against a wall for better support. This is more work for the man, especially if he need to lift and support his partner at the same time.

The Flying Buttress

The man lies on the bed on his back with legs open. Facing away from him, the woman climbs on top and extends her legs out to the back, whilst supporting herself with her forearms. This can take a bit of getting used to but it is worth working at it.

Chapter 11: Flexibility Positions

In reality both strength **and** flexibility go hand in hand, and there are historical interpretations and connections in the Kama Sutra that seem indicative of yoga influences – but essentially, whether it's strength or flexibility that defines a particular sexual position, the aim is the same: to increase stimulation and desire by pushing the body to its limit. The physiological effect of 'pushing the borders' is what is often referred to as a liminal reaction, that is, an experience that results in a spiritual and ecstatic realization.

Now, whether or not you have a religious awakening during sex aside, there is definitely an empirical basis for athletes undergoing a sense of altered or heightened awareness when pushed to the physical limit. So why shouldn't sex be able to accomplish the same thing? We've seen some strength-oriented sex positions, so let's take a look at someone's that require flexibility (and keep in mind that many of these are the sort you have to **practice** and work up to and are not necessarily for everyone!)

The Waterfall

We'll start off easy: the waterfall is similar to other variations we've seen and involves the man sitting on a chair with the woman propping herself on his lap to achieve penetration. The difference here is that the woman then bends backward down the man's legs so that her head is upside down. This can be very pleasurable for both partners since the man can stroke her stomach, breasts, and genital regions, while the woman allows herself to fall backward in the imitation of a waterfall – this mainly requires flexibility from the woman since she is essentially arching her back all the way back.

Reclining Pigeon

Not a terribly difficult position, this pose puts the woman on her back again. She brings up one knee, and then slides her opposing leg over top of it (you'll know you've got the position because of the pull in your gluteus maximums) – threading her arms under the leg on top, she uses both hands to clutch her other leg. By pulling up, she can manipulate the access to her vagina, and is a good equality technique – while the man approaches from the top and can initiate a rhythm, the woman is able to control the degree of friction by pulling up to enlarge the opening to the vagina.

> *Note this position is very good by itself at helping to relieve muscle tension in the rump area, but be careful about using it in sexual congress if you are stiff as it is very easy to pull this muscle.

The Shoulder Stand

Another position that seems right out of a yoga book this technique relies on the woman to have a strong back; she lies on her back, and the man stands on his knees. Gripping her by the waist he guides her up to his penis and, with her help, begins to enter her. The reason this position is so tricky is that it involves the man having to hold her up, and the woman is required to bend her back by almost 45 degrees in order to sustain the posture, which can leave you both sweating in no time at all.

The Mill Vanes

A very intimate and relatively moderate position, the mill vanes technique is a favorite of couples since it is a somewhat unusual position, yet manages to satisfy a considerable amount of clitoral stimulation. The woman lies on her back and then the man straddles over top of her (as one would do to initiate 69 oral sex). However, the man then leans all the way forward so that his penis can penetrate his partner – the angle of this coitus can be a fresh experience for both lovers but may require a few tries to get right. The man leans all the way forward on his stomach and the woman can help assist with this technique by folding her legs over the small of his back. For the woman, this can be a unique opportunity to get a glimpse of her lover's rump while having sex and can entice external stimulation by using her hands to caress his buttocks, thighs, or testicles.

The Bridge

Hailed as one of the more difficult Kama Sutra techniques to pull off – and usually not for long – the bridge makes a flexibility demand on the **man** this time. In a pose that will be familiar to yoga enthusiasts, the man creates an arc by leaning back so that his hands and feet are flat on the ground, and his stomach/chest is facing outwards. Just to achieve the base position can be strenuous, but once the man is ready, the woman kneels over top of his penis and inserts it into her vagina. She can then ride on top of him, stroking his chest or fondling his perineum – additionally, the positions can actually be reversed with the woman acting as the 'bridge.' In this case, the woman bends all the way back and arches her stomach toward the ceiling while the man gently clutches her by the waist to enter her. This can be amazingly seductive and arousing for the man for the same reason as the woman in the reversed position since he can stroke her stomach and breasts. For the woman, it is also easier since she doesn't have to worry about supporting her partner's weight as he is coming in from the side rather than straddling her.

> *Note it is a good idea for the woman to try and support as much of her weight as possible when the man is the 'bridge' in order to avoid injuring her partner or adding undue stress – this can sometimes be an issue with partners who are not equitable in height.

Fixing of the Nail

And we're back to the woman again; this position was even pointed out by Vatsyayana as requiring a special amount of practice given its acrobatic nature. The woman needs to bring one of her feet up to her head (think of someone trying to smell their own foot or bite their own toe), and then extend the other leg out in front of her. The man can then approach and enter her at her discretion – the result is one of the deepest penetrations, but requires a lot of flexibility. Because of its dynamics, it's also a good exercise for women with smaller or "tighter" vaginas because it will help ease open the vaginal passage and allow a smoother and more pleasant entrance of the penis.

The Crab Position

Another favorite, this one can be achieved by most women but still requires a degree of flexibility. The woman lies on her back again but this time brings up her legs and tries to place her feet on her abdomen. With her legs contracted and placed on her stomach, she can then push her arms under her knees to support them in that position – this opens up her vagina to allow her partner to penetrate. The benefit of this position is that it easily accommodated women who have all sizes of vaginas: for those with tighter entrances, the woman can simply open her arms and thereby spread her vagina wider. For women with larger vaginas, the opposite motion can be achieved by tucking in her arms and creating a smaller opening, which will increase friction and lead to a more pleasurable congress for both partners. This position is a nice balance between control, granting the man the 'upper' position by allowing him to guide and choose the rhythm and movement, but also allowing the woman to control the intensity of the sex.

The Rowing Boat

For those who want all the comfort and security of being able to face their partners with the added ability to maintain eye contact, then the Rowing Boat definitely fits the bill. This is a medium variety position in terms of flexibility, but offers some great support and requires good open communication (although it might take a few tries to get into a steady rhythm). Both partners face each other, and the man lies down to start – the woman may descend onto him until the penis is fully inserted, and then the man sits up again, so he is facing her. The man places his knees on the outside of her body, and she does the same, resulting in a sort of crossed leg situation. This is a very comfortable position, however, because partners can support themselves and the other by gripping their partner's legs. Since the knees of both partners are raised (and at chest level), it maximizes the amount of genital surface area for both – the man and the woman can then rock back and forth against each other, and while this position does not allow for a lot of external/internal movement of the penis in and out of the vagina, the opportunity to have both genital areas rubbing against one another makes this one of the more **stimulating** techniques for couples.

Dog Poses

Many yoga poses actually double as effective sexual postures as well (though don't tell Vatsyayana that). The dog poses – Downward Facing Dog being the most popular – involves the woman putting both her hands and feet flat on the ground and making a V with her body (the inverse of the Bridge); this allows easy access to the man who can enter her at her discretion. A variation of this is the Three-Legged Dog Pose which involves the woman lifting up one of her legs straight in the air so that it is lined up with her spine – think of trying to make the shape of the Greek letter Lambda with your body. Both positions require flexibility from the woman and give a significant amount of control and power to the man (which may become a preference for couples that enjoy domination scenarios).

The last variation on this we want to discuss is what it is called the Standing Straddle Forward Bend – more than just a mouthful; this could be an incredibly erotic position for either man or woman. In the traditional yoga pose, the woman in a standing position spreads her feet so that there is considerable width between them. Then, slowly, she bends over and grasps both her ankles. At this point, the man can come in behind her and control her hips with his hands. The exposure level of this position is very high, so it's very important that partners have already established a significant degree of trust.

Chapter 12: Relaxing Positions

While there is something to say about spicing up one's sex life by incorporating new and wild techniques and positions, at the same time we're not all acrobatics – in the same vein, that aforementioned 'spice' of life really is variety. In fact, the Kama Sutra is quick to point out that mastering a diverse array of different positions is ideal not only for keeping things interesting but also in terms of experimenting and opening one's self up sexually. The ability to try new things helps to broaden our horizons, and since you are entering this new realm with a partner, it can also be a very satisfying journey of self-discovery (and discovery of the other person).

That said, switching things up and allowing yourself to occasionally revert to simpler forms or positions, or at least ones that aren't super physically demanding, can give you and your partner a diverse repertoire of experiences to choose from. In previous chapters we've experimented with flexibility, strength, and gender-specific positions; now we'd like to end with some easy, relaxing sexual techniques.

Child Pose

Another borrowed pose from yoga, and a relaxing and spiritual cathartic one, is the child pose – this involves the woman sitting on her knees and then stretching forward with both her arms. This elegant and tender position allows the man to come in behind and enter her, and can also prostrate himself in a similar child pose, this time leaning forward **over her body**. This can be very relaxing and a good one to try even after orgasm as it helps to stabilize and activate the parasympathetic nervous system.

Ananda Balasana

Not strictly a sexual position either, this is a very easy and relaxing pose that can be pleasurable to the woman – the woman lies on her back and attempts to bring her feet up as high as she can, whereby she grabs them with her hands. Think of a baby trying to grab its toes. Luckily, most women can do this without much difficulty, and it doesn't require an undo amount of flexibility to achieve, but **does** produce a deep penetration all the way to the G-spot. Remember to keep eye contact with your partner to maintain this level of intimacy – the natural 'spring' created by the woman having her legs up in the air also produces an innate rhythm which can be pleasing.

Zen Pause Sex

A bit of a modern take on the idea of tantric sex, the Zen pause sex position is something you can integrate into a number of different positions, especially the more vigorous ones. In this position both partners are lying facing each other – we like to suggest this one when one or both of you are nearing climax. But instead of driving through with the orgasm, you both turn on your sides and hold each other (the man preferably being able to stay inside his partner as they collapse, and the woman wrapping or entwining her legs around him). This can help couples that have a hard time with endurance or premature ejaculation by giving you a chance to strengthen your resolve – holding each other and letting the orgasm dwindle, then building up speed and passion again can result in huge orgasms for both, and is a great technique for bringing multiple orgasms to the woman.

Close-Up, or Womb Embrace

This can be exercised as an actual sex position or as a comfortable and intimate position after orgasm. Both men and women lie in a classic spooning position but pull their legs up as far as they can to their chest – this makes the woman's rump extremely accessible to the man who can literally 'fold' around her form. At the same time, he can wrap his arms around her and kiss her neck and is a method we encourage men to adopt because it is a romantic and tender way to show a partner that they are loved. With so much body contact, it is a great way to open up one's energy and results in an extremely intimate blending – in the yoga tradition this could be compared to some methods of breath control like **pratiloman** that try to mimic a 'going back,' a way to relive what it was like to be in the womb. So you can see why this is such a powerful technique: the man in this context becomes like a metaphorical womb for his partner, nurturing an overwhelming sense of safety and security.

Reclining Lotus

If you haven't guessed yet, there are a lot of ways to improve or experiment with fundamental positions, and the Reclining Lotus can combine the intimacy level of the sitting Lotus with a somewhat more casual approach, especially if the woman is tired. The position involves the woman lying on her back and then crossing her legs as she would have done with the Lotus position, but this time the man enters her in a standard missionary style, with her legs pressing against his chest. Aside from giving the woman a break, the action of crossing her legs also produces a natural 'spring,' so this technique can create a very fluid sense of rhythm during congress.

Reclining Bend Angel

Another reclining position, this one is good to help increase endurance and extend the process of lovemaking. The woman lies on her back and brings both of her arms up above her head, holding both palms together. Not only does this help stretch out her abdomen, but it can also produce a very sexy curve in her posture – next she brings her legs up and attempts to touch both soles together. This involves forcing her knees down and outward, and therefore should only be attempted by a partner who is limber enough to do this without hurting herself (the knees should be able to touch the floor in this position). Finally, the man comes in and straddles over top of her, making sure not to disturb her legs so that they remain informed. With his knees on either side, he can dip into her vagina from a steep angle, creating an incredible amount of friction.

CONCLUSION

Throughout the last six chapters we've looked at a variety of elements related to Kama Sutra, everything from the philosophical framework that led to the development of the text (including the sacredness attached to the 'lingam' and 'yoni') to the importance of foreplay in both exciting and reproducing an environment and atmosphere of **trust**. The ability to share one's self – both emotionally and physically – is the hallmark of the Kama Sutra.

In our modern age, however, the Kama Sutra offers up another opportunity: to enliven our sex lives by engaging in positions that may seem unorthodox (and downright difficult!). But therein lies the beauty of it. Sex, like any other activity, and especially one that involves another person, requires **practice**. The ability to master a new sexual position is an enthralling moment for both partners.

Whether you're a new couple who are only beginning to explore each other's sexuality, or you've been together with someone for a long time, this book has hopefully opened your eyes to the exotic possibilities offered by tantric sex. But even though we've focused mainly on the physical components of lovemaking, it's useful (and healthy) to realize that any relationship must function on a number of levels in order to sustain itself and flourish.

We hope you've enjoyed – and take something away – from this book that you will be able to share and practice with your own partners. We also hope that no matter what, this book has at least demonstrated the necessity of keeping an open mind. After all, relationships are the most beautiful of adventures, and sex should be embraced with that same sensibility!

Chapter 13: Superior Sex Positions

Most people have a favorite sex position that is usually guaranteed to hit the spot just right. For most people, this is usually one of the positions designated for beginners.

However, there comes a time when beginner sex positions run the risk of becoming boring, monotonous, or unfulfilling. The longer a couple stays together, the more likely they are to want to try more thrilling sex positions to spice up their relationship. The great news is that there is an abundance of sexual positions that a couple can try ranging from beginner to advance to downright dangerous. Literally, there are thousands and thousands of sexual positions, and it can be quite an adventure for a couple to explore them.

One of the benefits of being more adventurous in your sex life and trying out more superior sexual positions is that it helps you last longer and prolong the journey to climax, which of course makes the final moments so much sweeter. Other benefits for trying out new sex positions include:

- **Targeting different pleasure points.** Different sex positions stimulate different parts of the body, and by trying out different positions, you can find pleasure points in your body that you did not even know existed before.

- **Different positions can incite different types of emotions.** A different position can change the way you perceive your relationship and your partner and can work as a catalyst to bring you two even closer.

- **Finding new ways to climax.** Experimenting with different positions allows you to better understand what feels good for your body and what can drive you harder and faster toward climax.

- **Increasing your sexual compatibility.** Sometimes, couples find that they are not as compatible as they would like with beginner sex positions, but more advanced positions make them feel more in tune with each other sexually.

Now, let's move into the spicier stuff. But first, it should be noted that these sex positions should not be tried out by beginners. If you have never been swimming before, you will not jump into the deep end of the pool without at least getting your feet wet, right? The same is true with sex. Start out slow and steady and over time, increase your repertoire to include more advanced positions.

Yoga for Advanced Sex Positions

To help with your transition into more advanced sex positions, it is a great idea to practice yoga so that there is less risk of injury and discomfort while allowing your body to move more smoothly into positions that require more physical fitness. Yoga is a great practice even if it is practiced for reasons other than improving your sexual function. It helps you become more aware of your body and teaches you to listen to the physical signs that your body sends you. It also allows you to become more in-tune with your mind so you can control your mental abilities.

The following yoga positions that will be discussed are particularly helpful to females.

The Bridge Pose

This yoga pose helps to strengthen your pelvic floor muscles, which lessens the likelihood of experiencing pain during sex for women. To achieve this yoga pose, lie on your back and bend both your knees. Your feet need to be positioned hip-width apart with your knees in line with your ankles. Keep your hands flat on the floor with your palms against the ground and your fingers spread. Lift your pelvis off the ground and allow your torso to follow but keep your shoulders and head on the floor. Hold this pose for 5 seconds before releasing.

The Happy Baby Pose

This pose is good for strengthening the lower back and gluteus. It also doubles as a great missionary position variation. To achieve this pose, lie on your back and bend your knees up toward your stomach while you exhale. When you inhale, reach to grab the inside of your feet and widen your knees. While pushing your heels upward, flex your feet and pull down with your hands to stretch.

The One-Legged Pigeon

Use this yoga pose to stretch and open up your hips. Tight hips can make sex uncomfortable and make it difficult to get into some sexual positions. To achieve this yoga pose, get on all fours on the floor. Pick up your right leg and place it in front of your body so that it is at a 90- degree angle away from your body. Stretch your left leg out behind so that the top of your foot faces downward and your toes are pointing backward. Lean forward on an exhale as you shift your body weight. Hold this pose for a few seconds then release and repeat on the other side.

Child's Pose

This pose helps you become more flexible as it opens up your hips. This pose is also a grounding one as it allows you to focus on resting and practicing breathing techniques which help melt away stress and anxiety. Enter this pose by kneeling on the floor and widening your knees until they are hip-width apart. On an exhale, lean forward and place your hands in front of you to stretch out. Allow your upper body to relax between your legs and touch your forehead to the floor. Hold this pose for 30 seconds to a few minutes.

The Cow Pose and the Cat Pose

These are two yoga poses being done in tandem to help you loosen up your spine, decrease stress levels, and get into the mood faster and easier. To get into this yoga position, start on all fours with your knees in line with your hips and your wrists below your shoulders. Your weight needs to be balanced evenly across your body, and your spine needs to be neutral.

Look up and inhale as you let your stomach curve toward the floor. Lift your chin and chest up as you stretch. On an exhale, tuck your chin back into your chest and draw your navel toward your spine as you round out your spine toward the ceiling.

Advanced Sex Positions

Standing Doggy Style

In this position, the couple stands with the woman facing away from the man. She bends over and anchors herself by hooking her hands around her ankles, calves or thighs. More flexible women are able to plant their hands on the floor. When the woman has achieved a stable position, the man penetrates her from behind and uses his hold on her hips to control the depth and intensity of his thrusts while helping her maintain her balance. In this position, the men can also stimulate the woman's clitoris.

The Cowgirl Lean Back

This position starts out like your traditional cowgirl position, but the woman does not remain on her knees. Instead, she moves her weight to the ball of her feet and squats over the man. The woman leans back to brace her hands on her partner's thighs and bounces up and down on his shaft. This position is great for G-spot stimulation and direct stimulation of the head of the man's penis.

The Sitting V

This position requires a woman to be more flexible. The woman needs to sit on a high bench or other flat surface while the man stands in front of her with his feet spread to maintain his balance. Their pelvises need to be aligned perfectly, and the woman needs to place her ankles on the man's shoulders so that her body makes the shape of a V. She can support herself by laying back on her arms, using a wall or by wrapping her arms around the man's neck. The man can support her by placing his hands around her back. The orgasms possible from this position are deeply stimulating because of the ability for strong thrusting and easy penetration.

X Marks the Spot

This position is similar to the Sitting V but differs because the woman lies on the flat surface. The man stands between her legs, lifts them into the air and crosses them to make an X. He can hold the woman's legs against him to keep her stable or she can balance her ankles on his shoulders. Because of the alignment of the pelvis, this is a great position for G-spot stimulation. Also, because of the crossing of the woman's legs, this position allows her core to feel even tighter around a man's penis.

The CAT Position

CAT stands for the coital alignment technique, and this advanced sex position is great for women who find it difficult to reach orgasm through sexual penetration alone. In this position, the man is more likely to reach her G-spot and stimulate her clitoris. To achieve this position, the couple starts out in missionary, and after penetration occurs, the man slides his pelvis a few inches higher than usual. He needs to keep his body flat against hers and rather than moving in and out of her, he needs to move up and down. The key to this position is that the couple remains pelvis to pelvis so that the base of the penis stimulates the woman's clitoris. The couple can take this position up a notch by placing a pillow under the woman while having the man use circular motions of his hips instead. The man can also grab the headboard and pull himself up and down.

Scissoring

This position is normally associated with sex between lesbians; however, heterosexual couples can engage in it as well. In this position, the woman lies on her side with her legs open and her knees slightly bent. The man is in a sitting position with his legs folded in an upside-down V. The two people allow their lower halves to meet at a near right angle. The man places his upper leg over her lower leg and his lower leg beneath hers so that he can shift closer for penetration to occur. There is a limited range of motion in this position, but the pleasure that can be had is astonishing. Both partners can stimulate the woman's clitoris, and because of the shallow nature of the thrust, the head of the man's penis is highly stimulated, which can build up to an earth-shattering orgasm.

The Waterfall

This is a variation of the popular cowgirl position, but the small variation packs a big punch in the pleasure that can be achieved. The man kicks this position off by laying on a couch or a bed with his head near the edge. The woman gets on top but instead of getting on her knees, she shifts her weight to the balls of her feet so that she is squatting over the man. Once she is in position, the man scoots closer to the edge of the bed until his head and shoulders slide onto the floor while his hips remain elevated. From that moment on, the woman has complete control over the intensity, depth, and speed of hip thrusts. Since her hands are free, she can also use them to stimulate her partner and herself.

The Double Decker

This position is a variation of the woman on top position and entails having both parties lie on their backs with the woman on top of the man facing away from him. She leans back and keeps herself propped up with her elbows. The man spreads his thighs while she places hers between his. When their pelvises are aligned, penetration is possible. This position is great for dirty talk as well since the man's mouth is right next to the woman's ear.

Sex Positions for Experts

The sex positions that will be discussed in this section can be labeled as dangerous. They are physically challenging and should be tried at your own risk.

The Advanced High Squeeze

In this position, the woman lies on her back and plants her feet on the man's chest. The man is in a kneeling position and her buttocks are lifted to meet his pelvis. The challenge in this position is that the woman is supported by her upper back, and the reward is G-spot stimulation. This is also a good position for men who have a foot fetish since they can nibble on the woman's toes while the two get it on.

The Wheelbarrow

In this position, the woman is on her hands and knees and a man stands up. He then grabs hold of her ankles and pulls her lower body off the floor until she is completely supported by him. He fits himself between her spread thighs. Many adventurous couples love this position because there is something simultaneously animalistic and acrobatic about it. Some couples add even more spice to it by making the woman move about using her hands, which are planted on the floor. The man follows behind and continues to thrust.

The Pretzel

In this position, both parties start out by doing a crab walk, which is the position of having both their hands and feet planted firmly on the ground with their stomach facing the ceiling. The couple has their heads facing in opposite directions, and the woman moves until she is above her partner so that her pelvis is directly above his. She lowers herself so that she can be penetrated by him. For this position to be successfully pleasurable, both partners need to have good core, leg, and arm strength.

The Arch

In this position, the woman gets into the crab walk position and the man kneels between her thighs while facing her. The man helps support the woman by placing his hands underneath her buttocks. The woman needs to have good core, leg, and arm strength to maintain this position, but the tradeoff is that her G-spot is stimulated and her partner can also use one hand to touch her clitoris.

Reverse Missionary

In this position, the man lies on this back and brings his knees up to his chest. His penis juts out from between his thighs and the woman squats above him so that her vagina is aligned with his penis. She lowers herself to be penetrated and controls the depth and intensity of the strokes as she is in a superior position. This position can be challenging for the man since pressure is being applied to the back of his thighs. This position is great for developing intimacy in a relationship.

Chapter 14: Sitting Sex Positions

Sex is a desire of enjoying life with full intent and passion. This demands more variations to repel boringness and enthusiast both partners. One of these variations is sitting family sex positions. They allow the male partner to sit on a chair or sofa and make room for the female to sit on his lap and give up her body to his desires. The female partner allows him to take over and control the movement with the intensity of penis inclusion inside the vagina and anal hole. Penis inclusion in the holes may be straight, with enormous rubbing and stimulating clitoral rubbing, or curvy. with the weight of the ass involved. Moreover, these positions allow intense exposure of the body, making it viable for both to kiss and lick the bodies, especially boobs, and feel the heat of the moment. Going harsher to your lady with fast inclusions could double the joys and bring about immense sexual experiences. This sex position family is the best choice for those who need to relax to get the top of pleasure. Man erection will be easier and stronger, while women will easily reach the top of their sensual feelings.

Kneeling Lotus

When it comes to best mobility actions, the lotus sex positions are tried and enjoyed a lot due to their adventurous rides. In this position, the man sits on his ass, folding his legs and making room for his lady on his lap. His fists are placed backward, eventually using a pillow to make it more comfortable. The woman, being on top, sits on his lap by opening her legs, making enough room for man's penis and folding her knees backward. On the other hand, the man's body is inclined backward with his fists touching the ground. The woman puts her hands on his shoulders, making him realize her body and her assets. Both the partners are lying face-to-face and immense kissing and licking experience is vitalized. The best way to accomplish and feel enthusiastic in this position is by doing it faster. This is purely intimate and adventurous sex as it allows man's penis to go inside her vagina by rubbing her lips and turning sex into a mild experience. It exposes her whole body to her man and intimates the best spanking and licking experience.

Sitting Bull

Being another position of sitting family sex positions, it carries more adventure with higher intensity and greater affection. The woman sits beside her partner, on the floor, and allows him to freely go inside her vaginal by rubbing and squeezing her pelvis and opening her for his penis. It offers more comfort, but with a difficulty of more fast mobility. Mobility is not as easy in this position as in other sitting positions. The man also sits beside his partner with face-to-face contact and allows kissing, licking, and breasts sucking with its full intent. On the other hand, the woman licks his body to increase her mildness. This way, both partners can go wild, crazy and allow rough sex with strong emotional attachments and deeper physical contacts. This position becomes more enjoyable if the woman leans back a little, using her arms and legs to generate penetration distance. The harsher you go with your partner, the better it will be and more rubbing, with strong clitoral stimulation, guaranteed. As a result, satisfaction roses higher and higher.

Squatting Bull

Another enthusiastic experience of sitting style sex positions, while going with the woman sitting, in a squat position, on man's lap and enjoying realistic and simulative sex. Man, with straight legs, is lying down sitting beside his lady, allowing her to ride and explore the beauties of sex. Both partners are face-to-face, experiencing enormous kissing, licking and rubbing experiences with strong vaginal intercourse. The woman rubs her pussy by using her hand continuously while indulging deep in sex and going harsh by fastening the in and out of the penis. Most female partners find it more comfortable to carry along and can have a spanking posture a little long. On the other hand, man is likely to love this position if he goes deep inside her vaginal hole by lifting his hips a little and making it easy for him to move faster, satisfying both. This, by going wild, could guarantee more quickly cumming of the woman and double her joys with more vicious satisfactions. Going deep would turn sex into a mild experience.

Planted Bull

Another joyous sitting position and enthusiastic for its mobility and easiness. The planted bull variation brings the woman's feet to the floor and allows her to let her body on her partner, giving him full access to her vagina and anal hole with the choice of either going deep inside the anal hole or rubbing more by going curvy inside of the vagina. The harsher you go on with your partner, the more satisfying it will be for her and more quickly she will offload from her cum. Another approach to making it intense is controlled movement by the woman with a gentle push off with his legs and pull back using the man's thighs. This position exposes her whole body and makes it more viable for those who love full exposure and immense kissing experiences. The man could easily suck her boobs to enjoy the heat of the moment. If this position seems uncomfortable for you because of rubbing or strong stimulation, you can stick to rolling the hips or could use it as a resting way. The experience could be a lot better by putting pillows beneath both of you.

Lying Bull

Sex, if adopted to fulfill desires and done more frequently, will turn into a boring one. But trying different positions from time to time will make it more pleasant, joyous and plausible, especially for the female partner. These positions will draw pleasures, come to ecstasy and make the full of it by indulging both partners deeply. In lying bull position, the man sits on the floor, the woman is down on her knees and fully leans forward with her arms overhead, overstretched and legs rested on man's legs, with the man who caresses or slaps, with her accordance, her ass and goes curvy in the vaginal and anal hole. Man's legs are driven apart with the woman on her lap, giving him full exposure of her holes. The men who love to watch every inch going inside her holes will love this position as it explores and widens every angle of going inside. The more they push, the more it goes inside. For experienced couples, more feast is in the form of licking the holes and, for woman, sucking his cock and balls.

Lap Dance

Another sitting fiesta is the famous lap dance sex position. This is quite amazing when it comes to its peak. It offers flexibility, fastness and rubbing together with strong clitoral stimulation as well as exposure of female's back to her male partner. In this style of sex, the woman has her legs positioned inside the men. This guarantees a bit controlled penetration but, with a gentle push from the male, it could go deeper inside her holes. The deeper you go, the more enthusiastic it will be. But this position may come out herder on legs, as the whole weight of the body is on legs, with tilted ass and leaned on the man's penis. It may stretch muscles a bit too. But going smoother will solve the question. Try using different exposures like going front to back, side to side, back to front and much more. The best thing is that it allows anal gaping and deep penetration in the anal hole that is way more joyous for some males and females too.

Lap Dance 180

The lap dance 180 is quite similar to lap dance position and the only difference is the spinning of the woman towards the man, lying on her lap with face-to-face exposure. The more she comes near her man, the more joy it will be for both the partners. This position allows her to put her arms around his neck. indulging him to suck her boobs and kiss her everywhere on upper parts of the body while the man, having his arms on her buttocks, pushes her forward to make deep penetration possible. The man sits on a chair and relaxes by going deep inside her holes. Both holes are easily accessible with the option of going curvy inside the anal hole. The vaginal hole may not encounter enough rubbing as the vagina is right above the penis and allows frictionless inclusion. The woman with widened legs may suffer discomfort and less mobility. But this could be solved by using a sturdy chair to avoid accidents. Being on face-to-face with the partner could enthusiast the mildness and drive both partners into the craziness.

Squatting Lap Dance

This is another amazing position in the class of sitting style sex positions. It is full of adventure and enthusiasm. In this squatting position of the lap dance, the woman squats on the same surface on which the man is sitting on. Try to do this position on a stable chair with armrests to guarantee comfort and plausible joys. If a table chair isn't available, try using man's legs and leaning forward. This position allows the touching of the bodies and intense licking experiences together with sucking and kissing. This could be done a lot better if he holds her back or her waist. The man can lick and kiss her waist too. On the other hand, the woman can allow him easy access to both the holes and delight the experience of the sex. Being on top of his lap, the vaginal and anal hole is right above the penis. Therefore, it will drive frictionless inclusion and could be controlled by the woman, sitting on the penis up to the extent where length is bearable.

Folded Lap Dance

Another joyous position within the class of sitting sex positions is the folded lap dance. In this position, the man sits on a chair, or any other horizontal place, making room for the woman to sit on his lap. The woman, lying in his lap, puts her legs on his shoulders by folding her knees, making it a folded lap dance. This allows exposure of her breasts and the front side of the body, which faces closer enough to kiss and develop the heat with joy. By indulging in each other's body, the experience could be a lot more joyous and sensational. Man can go deep inside her vaginal hole but will find it difficult to go inside her anal hole as it allows curvy inclusion with enough resistance due to lying right above the penis. But woman, by leaning backward on his hands, could allow anal gaping and deep penetration in the anal hole, allowing him to taste the anal hole and make a viable ground for anal sex.

Chapter 15: Standing Sex Positions

Couples do not usually like standing sex positions because of the effort that they require. Orgasm is harder to achieve in these positions, and oral and manual stimulations are not easy to do either.

What many couples do not know is that standing sex positions can provide sheer excitement and explosive orgasms.

First, couples can experience increased libido as a result of increased excitement, which ultimately results in more pleasure. The reason is the uniqueness of the experience, which makes sex more memorable (especially for couples who will try standing sex positions for the first time).

Second, many standing sex positions allow the woman to stretch her vaginal walls and clitoris in unusual ways. This gives her a different kind of pleasure. Moreover, the man can also penetrate her in unusual angles, which stimulates his penis in ways that are very different from what he usually does (when compared to the common sex positions and strokes in masturbation).

Lastly, standing sex positions actually open a lot of the couple's pleasure spots to oral and manual stimulation, such as the face, neck, nape, breasts, shoulders, back, hips, and buttocks. With proper balance, the couple can just kiss and grope each other while the man thrusts in and out until both of them reach orgasm.

Give your sex life a new kind of twist with these steamy standing sex positions.

12. Dancer Sex Position

How to do it: Most ballroom dancers like doing this position as their finale pose, hence, the name. This time, the couple will still be dancing only to a more sensual rhythm that unites their bodies.

The couple stand facing each other. The man grabs the woman's leg and raises it to his hips. She then wraps her arms around his neck for support while he penetrates her. This can also be done with her back against the wall for better balance.

Pros: She also experiences clitoral stimulation, depending on how tight their bodies are against each other. Eye-to-eye contact is also consistent until the couple reach orgasm.

Cons: The position can be tiring for her since she will be balancing on only one foot. The man also needs to be strong enough to support their combined weight.

13. Ballerina Sex Position

How to do it: This position is a more extreme version of the Dancer Sex Position. Like in the last position, the couple stands facing each other. Instead of raising the woman's leg up to the man's hips or waist, she stretches her leg all the way up to his shoulder. This is more difficult, but the greater difficulty only highlights the sensation of every thrust.

Pros: This will be very intense for the woman as this stretches her vaginal walls, making them look and feel tight. This position also opens up her clitoris and breasts for non-stop manual stimulation.

For him, the penetration will give him more intense pleasure as her vagina is tighter. He will also have access to all of her pleasure spots, especially the clitoris and breasts.

Cons: The great amount of flexibility required for this position may not be suitable for all women. Furthermore, she might find it hard to balance on one foot, especially if the man is too tall for her height.

14. Tree Climbing Sex Position

How to do it: This sex position is more extreme than the other recently discussed positions as it requires the man to carry all the weight while initiating penetration and oral stimulation.

The man stands straight with his legs apart for better balance. The woman then climbs on him by straddling him by the waist. Her legs should be locked around his waist and her arms locked around his neck. To penetrate, he lifts her a little by grabbing her butt.

To reduce the level of difficulty, he can push her against the wall or raise her legs up to his back (lowering her legs will only make her heavier).

Pros: The difficulty of this sex position highlights the sensation that both the man and the woman can feel. The rarity of this position also makes many couple more excited when performing it.

Cons: The man needs to be strong enough to balance and carry the woman while thrusting. Manual stimulation will also be limited as the couple's hands will be busy keeping balance.

Chapter 16: Balanced Positions

These positions are called "balanced" because both you and your woman practically need to do the same thing in order to achieve synchronicity in movements. Performing these positions is a special time to feel that you and your partner are equal on bed.

Chair Riding Position

You need two chairs as both you and your woman have to perform this on top of them. Keeping the chairs together while penetrating is one part of making it exciting.

Have the chairs face each other with the smallest gap possible. Sit down on one chair and open your legs so that your feet are resting on the other. Now, ask her to sit down as well with both legs opened but still positioned between yours. Your penis should be in close contact to make penetration easy and deep.

Thrusting back and forth is more difficult, so you may want to thrust up and down while she moves downwards and upwards (so you meet halfway). This will also prevent the chairs from separating, and both of you falling down.

Octopus Position

This one is similar to the chair riding position, but it is performed on a bed instead. Like the latter, you sit and open your legs to accommodate her between yours. The difference though is that in this position, her ankles are placed on your shoulders. Her raised angle makes penetration deeper and more stimulating.

To make it even more exciting, you can let her sit on your lap entirely while she supports her weight with her arms. Thrusting can come from both of you, but you have to be careful in moving her on your lap to avoid breaking your penis.

Jellyfish Position

It is probably the most tiring in this set of "sexercises," but the sensation it brings is intense and the position is extremely intimate. Both you and your woman need to have a good sense of balance and strength to perform it, though.

Start by squatting as you put the weight of your butt on your ankles and calves. She then needs to straddle you without losing her balance on the floor or bed. Both of you are in a tight position by now, so you have to embrace each other tightly as you rock back and forth.

Your lower bodies will take the toll, but it can be really explosive for her as the sensation of every thrust is contracted by muscle tensions.

35. Scissors Position

Imagine a scissor whose two blades cross each other as they lock in place. That is essentially what you are trying to do here.

Lie on your side so that one leg is supporting your body while the other is free to rise and open your penis to her vagina. Ask her to also do the same so that both of you are locked between each other's legs. You have a perfect alignment of organs in this position and can thrust in complete unison.

Sockets Position

This is a variation of the Scissors Position, but instead of doing it while lying on your side, you do it while lying face up. You can do it from the Scissors Position or from another position on the bed. Open your legs so that one of hers can go between you. Enter her by slowly pointing your penis downwards (towards her vagina), so your thrusting motions will also be in that direction.

It can be a little uncomfortable to you at first because your penis is bent downwards, but the pressure it gives to her vaginal walls can be quite intense. Just be careful when you thrust as the penis is not flexible.

Poles Apart Position

This position is an excellent way to stimulate her G-spot without having to perform deep penetration. As the term implies, both of you will be lying in straight but in the opposite direction just like poles apart.

Lie on your side facing the same direction as in the Spoon Position. However, instead of having both of your heads on the same side, one of you needs to change side so that both of your heads are now opposite directions. Your penis and her vaginal opening should be in complete alignment and both of you need to be lying as straight as possible.

Bumper Cars Positions

This position comes with an unusual rear entry, but the angle of penetration gives intense sensation, especially to the woman whose stimulation of vaginal wall is quite different. Nevertheless, you might find it uncomfortable at first as your penis will be thrusting while pointing downwards.

Ask her to lie face down with legs open to accommodate your penis. Do the same but with your head in the opposite direction. Slide your penis inside until you are comfortable to move.

Ex Sex Position

This is similar to the Bumper Cars Position, but your woman will be lying on her back instead to make it easier for you to penetrate, thrust, and gyrate. As she lies down, position yourself on top of her but with your head in the opposite direction. Your penis will be slightly bent downwards, but it should be more comfortable than in the Bumper Cars Position.

Chapter 17: Sensual Positions

Sensual positions are extremely emotional and generally come from a more loving place in the heart. Emotional romantics tend to love sensual positions as they allow them to get physical stimulation as well as emotional stimulation which heightens the experience and makes it even easier for them to have a mind-blowing orgasm. If your partner is an emotional romantic, you will want to include sensual sex in your experience. Remember, not every experience needs to be sensual and not every experience needs to be **only** sensual. It is perfectly okay and even normal to mix it up.

Many people feel as though sensual sex is only the missionary position, but this is not true. There are actually many different positions that can be sensual for you and your partner to enjoy together. While missionary is one of them, there are many others you can consider. The following 20 positions will add a sensual element to your sexual experience.

The Rocking Horse

This position is an elaborated version of the missionary style. It is a female-on-top position that allows the female partner to have near-total control over the movements. This position allows both partners to lovingly gaze at each other or cuddle each other as they make love. Because of the set-up of the position, the man can also take over and have control over the movements as well. Please click the link below to see the Rocking Horse Position.

Him: Put your arms out behind you and lean back on them as you sit up. Your legs can either be straight out in front of you, knees up, or crossed. If you are controlling the movement, you may want to have your knees bent for leverage, but otherwise sit however feels comfortable for you.

Her: Sit on top of your man with a leg on either side of his hips. You should be on your knees, using your shins as leverage to help you with movements. However, you can sit in any way that feels comfortable to you and your partner. From this position, you can cradle your man's head, look into his eyes, or even put his face on your chest if that feels comfortable.

The Slide

This is another girl-on-top position, but both partners are able to have more control over the movements in this one. Still, because of the position, the female will have slightly more control than the male when it comes to thrusting. This position is very close to missionary but has a slight twist on it which makes it have a unique feeling.

Him: You want to lie on your back with your legs out straight. Once your partner is on top of you, you can use your hands to caress her back or bum, or you can even hold her face and kiss her as she rides you.

Her: You want to lay down on top of your man, keeping your legs straight out as well. While you can sit in whatever position you like, the straighter you keep your legs, the more your g-spot will be stimulated with this position.

The Nirvana

This is a man-on-top variation of missionary that gives him a greater opportunity to reach the g-spot and bring her to climax. It also allows the partners to look into each other's eyes and have an emotional experience brought into the bedroom. Please click the link below to see the Nirvana Position.

https://bit.ly/2FhnQDi

Her: You want to lay down on your back with your legs straight out. For the best g-spot action make sure that your thighs are pressed together, and you do not spread your legs.

Him: You should get on top of your partner now and put one knee on either side of her thighs, helping her keep her legs together. Then, enter her from the front. You can prop yourself up on your hands or elbows to help you from crushing her. From here you can look into her eyes, kiss her, or even cuddle your face into her neck.

The Padlock

This is a saucier position that is still easy for average couples to experience. It involves the use of a surface that is roughly waist-high for the male partner, so you can use your bed, a table, a countertop, or anything else that provides the right height for the male in the relationship.

Her: You want to sit on top of the waist-height surface and lean back on your arms. Once he has entered you, you can adjust your lean-to find where it feels the best for you. If you want, you may wish to use a cushion or blanket underneath you so that it is less pressure on your tailbone and spine during this position. Once he enters you, you want to wrap your legs around him and lock your heels between his thighs.

Him: Once your partner has gotten comfortable on the surface, you want to lean in and enter her. You can use your hands behind her hips to help you get leverage for thrusting. She will then lock her feet between your thighs, so be sure to stand with your feet spread so she can create the "padlock."

The Ascent to Desire

While this may not be effective for all couples, it will be a wonderful position for couples where the male partner can easily lift the female partner. This position allows the female to develop a sense of trust in the male as he is holding her up and she must rely on him not to drop her. It is also an excellent position for maximizing g-spot and clitoral stimulation. Please click the link below to see the Ascent to Desire Position.

Him: You are simply going to stand and lift your partner up. You can use her thighs or bum to hold her so that you do not drop her. It may be easier to have her sitting on the bed or another waist-high surface at first so that you can enter her and lift her easier. Once she is lifted, you can begin thrusting.

Her: As he lifts you, use your arms to hold onto his shoulders. You can lean back slightly to maximize the pleasure you experience. Be sure to lean slowly so that you do not throw your man off balance! Let your legs swing freely with this one; it is all about relaxing into the pose for it to work.

The Suspender

This is another standing position where the man holds the female. This time, the position is slightly different, and the female is more responsible for holding herself up. Based on the structure of the position, it makes it easier for the female to orgasm from g-spot stimulation. It is also easier for the male to keep his balance and maximize the pleasure from the position.

Him: You are going to pick your lady up, rest her over you and then lean back against a wall. The support of the wall will help you keep your balance and will make thrusting significantly easier. You can hold your hands under her bum to help her keep her balance as you are thrusting.

Her: When he lifts you up, you are going to want to hold his shoulders or neck for support. If you want to get more energy out of the movement, you can put your feet on the wall behind him and push off of it for momentum. This will help build up the sensation of the position and make it more pleasurable for the both of you. It will also take some of the work off of him.

The Sexy Spoon

Simple spooning can be turned into passionate, romantic sex with the sexy spoon. This position allows you to cuddle while having sex. Because of the nature of this position, your bodies meld together perfectly making it a highly sensual position that can have an increased pleasure for both parties. Please click the link below to see the Sexy Spoon Position.

https://bit.ly/2UE1a5n

Her: This position is easiest for you. You simply want to lay on your side with your knees bent, so that your man can access you from behind. In essence, you are the "little spoon" in this position.

Him: You are going to be the big spoon, coming up with your girl from behind. You can cuddle her, just as you would in regular spooning, and then enter her from behind. If you want to increase her pleasure, put your knees together between her legs so that hers are spread apart. You can then hug her or cup her breasts while you thrust.

The Reverse Spoon

This reverse spoon position has both partners facing one another as you have sex. It is almost like a missionary on the side, only a little different. Both lovers will need to put in the effort for the thrusting to work. It is a very sensual position that has you very close to one another, touching with virtually every part of your body. Please click the link below to see the Reverse Spoon Position.

https://bit.ly/2Ji7BtT

Him: You are going to lay on your side facing your partner. You want to be leaning back slightly so that you can get leverage to thrust her. You can put a pillow behind your back for added support if the lean is too uncomfortable for you. Alternatively, your woman can put her leg behind your back and hold you up with her leg.

Her: You are going to mount your man from the side, putting your leg over his hip and behind his back. To help him out, you can put your knee down behind his back and use your leg to support him in the position. From there, you can cuddle him while you both move to thrust.

The Glowing Juniper

This position requires a little more flexibility, but it is still an incredibly comfortable position to enter. It is also highly enjoyable for many women as it helps the man hit directly on the g-spot, making penetration much more enjoyable. It also allows the man to enter deeper than other positions, meaning he will get maximum pleasure from this position, too.

Him: You are going to sit with your legs straight out in front of you, spread open so that your woman can lay between them. You are not in charge of the thrusting in this position, so this will be more of a pleasure pose for you.

Her: You are going to lay down with your back between your man's legs and your legs wrapped around either side of his chest. Your feet should be on the floor or bed behind your partner. Then, you can use your legs as leverage to push off of your man. This gives you full control over penetration depth and speed.

The Kneel

This face to face position is vertical, so both partners are upright. You are not standing for this position, however, which makes it a unique and fun pose to try out. Both partners get full control over motion and momentum, meaning that as much or as little energy can be put into the thrusting motions of the position.

Him: You are going to be sitting up on your knees, holding your lady in front of you.

Her: You are going to want to sit on your knees with one on either side of your man's thighs. Then, you can mount him and hug him as well as you both thrust.

The Rock N Roller

This position combines the pleasures of face to face positions and face to back positions. It is an extremely easy move to get into and can be done by virtually anyone. This position allows for her g-spot to be stimulated while he gains a deeper penetration.

Her: You are going to lay on your back with your legs in the air. Once your man gets into position, you will rest them on his shoulders. You can use a pillow under your head as well as under your tailbone if you need extra support to keep this position comfortable for you. The pillow under the tailbone can also make it easier for your man to get deeper penetration.

Him: You are going to scoot in and enter your lady while she puts her legs over your shoulders. This position will put you in total control so you can go as deep as you want and you control the movement. Always be sure to start slowly and move at her pace, as entering too deeply too quickly can cause pain and ruin the moment for you two.

The Amazon

This position is a simple position that involves a chair and allows you and your partner to gain a deeper entry and a great sensual experience. It is a woman-on-top position that gives her the most control over the movement, but he can contribute if he wants to as well.

Him: You are going to sit on a chair with your knees out in front of you and your feet flat on the floor. When she mounts you, you can hug her, hold her bum to gain some control over the movements and help her out, or you can place them anywhere else that feels comfortable and natural for you.

Her: You are going to mount your man, putting one leg on either side of the chair. You will want to have your feet planted firmly on the floor as this is what will give you leverage for your position. You can hug him or place your hands wherever feels comfortable. If you need more leverage to help with movement, you might consider holding the back of the chair and using your arms to help pull you up with each bounce.

The Super 8

This is a spiced-up version of the traditional missionary position. It is an extremely easy man-on-top position that adds pleasure and comfort to the experience. Because of the position's structure, it allows for maximum eye-gazing and sensuality to be added to the experience.

Her: You are going to lay on your back on the bed, using a pillow under your head for comfort if need be. When your man mounts you, you can then wrap your legs behind his knees so that he can get a deeper penetration.

Him: You are going to mount your lady like you would missionary style, only instead of having your legs around hers, they are going to be between hers. You can then rest up on your hands so that you are well above her, allowing you to gaze into her eyes while you are thrusting.

Curled Up

This position is like a variation of the Rock N Roller. You are going to get the best of both face to face and face to back facing positions, allowing you the opportunity to get deeper penetration and sensual eye-gazing in. Of course, from the nature of this position, it has maximum g-spot action, so you can guarantee that both are going to get great pleasure from this position!

Her: You are going to lay on your back with your legs up in the air. When your man mounts you, you want to put your feet on his chest, curling your knees up into your chest. This position takes away virtually all of your control over the movement but allows for deep entry and great g-spot stimulation.

Him: You are going to scoot up behind your girl and enter her as though you are entering her from behind. When you do, she will put her feet on your chest. You can then put your hands next to her shoulders and thrust at your own free will. Remember, she does not have any control in this position so listen to her cues to ensure that the position is enjoyable for both of you.

The Proposal

This position gives a whole new purpose to getting down on one knee. Only with this position, you are both getting down on one knee. It may be awkward for some, but for those who can get into this position and maximize movements, they will gain significant amounts of pleasure from this position.

Him: You are going to get down on one knee. When she gets down in front of you, you can cup her bum to get more control over the movement. While she will have control over this movement, it will primarily be you who is getting the thrusting action in. She will be rocking her hips to meet your thrusts.

Her: Get down on one knee in front of your man, with the same knee forward. It should result in each of you having one leg up next to each other's hip on the same side. You should put your foot on the other side of his shin so that you can get a good locking action going between your bodies. Hug him for support, and as he thrusts, you can rock your hips to meet his action.

Blossoming Lotus

This is a sitting down position that looks a lot like sitting cross-legged. It is a female-on-top position, and because of the angle the man's legs will be at, the female must take control of this one. It is a very pleasurable position and allows the lady to choose penetration depth and speed.

Him: You are going to sit down with your ankles crossed on the ground. If the pressure of someone on your lap hurts your ankles, you can also sit with the bottoms of your feet touching.

Her: You are going to mount your man and sit with your feet behind him. This position relies more on rocking than on bouncing, so you can touch the bottoms of your feet together as well if it is comfortable. Find the position that feels natural to you that allows you to rock back and forth while still getting enough pleasure from the position.

The Sphinx

This is a position that allows the man to enter from the back. It is a highly pleasurable position that gives the woman the opportunity to have control in the movements as well. While she will likely not take full control, she can rock her hips back to meet each thrust.

Her: Start by sitting on your hands and knees. Then, squat your pelvis to the bed and bend your arms so that you are resting on your forearms. You should look as though you are in the same pose as a sphinx. When he thrusts you, you can rock your hips back to meet his movements.

Him: You can enter like you are in doggy position, or you can lay with your legs straight out behind you and thrust that way. Lay in any way that feels most comfortable to you for this position. You have the most control so that penetration will be up to you for this one.

The Side Kick

This is another position that allows the man to enter from the back and gives him full control over movements. It is a very sensual pose that is highly relaxing for the female. This position allows great clitoris stimulation and is easy for the man to get leverage on the thrusting as well.

Her: You want to lay on your stomach with your legs straight out. You can also bend one knee up to the side if you prefer, as this will give you added clitoris stimulation. This position is meant to be relaxing for you, so there is not much you need to do, besides relax completely into the position.

Him: You are going to come up behind your lady on your knees, entering her from behind. You can hold her hip so that you get more leverage on thrusting, which will give you the ability to penetrate at any depth or speed you desire. You can also practice moving your hips around a little so that you gain g-spot stimulation as well, maximizing her pleasure from this position.

The Waterfall

This position does require balance and flexibility, but it can be highly sensual and extremely stimulating when done correctly. The waterfall is a woman-on-top position that requires the man to make all of the efforts in thrusting. Please click the link below to see the Waterfall Position.

Him: You are going to sit on a chair with your knees out in front of you. When your lady mounts you, you are going to hold her back to allow her to lay back on your legs. You will need to support her to ensure she doesn't fall during this position. Once she is laying back, you can begin to thrust.

Her: You are going to mount your man like you do in the Amazon pose, but this time you are going to lay back over his lap and pull your knees up in the air. Your entire body should be completely supported by his, giving him total control over the movements in this position.

The Right Angle

This is an extremely easy position that gives great stimulation and pleasure to both parties. It can be accomplished by anyone and can be done virtually anywhere in your home or anywhere else. Additionally, you can customize this position to maximize pleasure by giving different stimulation to various areas of the sexual organs.

Her: You are going to lay back on any surface that is roughly waist-high for your man. If there isn't one, you can lay on any surface that would be waist-high if he were on his knees. When he enters you, you can put your feet on his chest, your legs over his shoulders, your legs around his back, or anywhere else that feels comfortable for you.

Him: You are going to enter your girl from between her legs. Depending on what surface she is on, you may be able to stand, or you may have to go down on your knees. If you are on your knees, you might consider putting a pillow beneath them for added support and comfort. You will get a full-body view of her, so you can gaze in all of her beauty while thrusting.

Chapter 18: Top 15 Sex Positions & How to do Them

The Missionary 180

This position puts a spin on the traditional missionary position, but it requires the man to be flexible! The woman needs to lay down on her back with her legs spread apart. The man then lies on top, but with his head down towards her feet – his legs should then be on either side of her body. Once in position, the man should carefully push his penis downwards and penetrate his partner. Get comfortable and perform upward and downward thrusts.

Safety advice

This position requires the man to have a very flexible penis – make sure he is comfortable before committing to the position! There is a risk of him straining his penis's suspensory ligaments. If he does feel any significant pain you should consider leaving the position behind and finding something better suited and comfortable. When entering the position, the woman should be careful not to pull hard on the penis while guiding it inside her.

The Bumper Car

This is an extreme sex position that allows for deep penetration. This is great if you require G-spot stimulation to reach orgasm. Again, this position requires penile flexibility, so make sure the man is comfortable with the position. Start with the woman laying down on her stomach with her legs wide open and straight out. The man should then lie down on his stomach, with his legs open and straight out. He must be facing in the opposite direction. Afterward, the man reverses back towards his partner so his thighs are resting over hers. He needs to do this until he is able to point his penis towards his partner's vagina. Then penetrate slowly.

Safety Tips

This position requires penile flexibility. If you want to find out if the man's penis is flexible enough, have him stand against a wall. Pull his penis gradually down. If the penis is able to point directly down to the ground without causing pain then you should be fine to perform this position, but still, be careful. The woman should stay still when the man is initially penetrating her. The woman should wait while he finds the most comfortable position and angle to thrust without injury.

Man Trap

This is a variation of the missionary position. The woman should lie back on a bed in the missionary position and have the man lay on top. As he begins to thrust, the woman can wrap her legs around him and have more control over the speed and pace of sex.

This is great if you just want some simple sex. You can put little twists on the move like arching the back for better stimulation. Wrapping the legs around the man will also get him going a lot faster!

Safety Tips

This position can cause a lot of strain on the female's lower back, so make sure support is provided by using a pillow or cushion! Be sure to ask whether your partner is comfortable and not in any pain at any point and don't be ashamed if you need to say something because *you* are uncomfortable!

The Lustful Leg

Start by standing close and facing each other. The woman should have one leg on the bed and the other on top of the man's shoulder, whilst wrapping her arms around his back and neck for support. Then he should carefully penetrate.

Once in position, this is a great move that feels fantastic! It does, however, require some endurance.

Safety Tips

This position requires penile flexibility, else there is a risk of the man straining his suspensory ligaments!

 If you want to find out if the man's penis is flexible enough, have him stand against a wall. Pull his penis gradually down. If the penis is able to point directly down to the ground without causing pain then you should be fine to perform this position, but still be careful.

The woman should stay still when the man is initially penetrating her and guide the penis to the vagina. The woman should wait while he finds the most comfortable position and angle to thrust without injury.

The Deckchair

The male should sit on the bed with his legs stretched out and his hands behind him to support his own weight. He should lean back and bend his elbows slightly. The female should then lie back on a pillow facing him and put her feet up on to his shoulders. She can then move her hips forwards and back and begin having sex.

This is an amazing position for very deep penetration for G-spot stimulation.

Safety Tips

This position can cause a lot of strain on the female's lower back, so make sure support is provided by using a pillow or cushion! Be sure to ask whether your partner is comfortable and not in any pain at any point and don't be ashamed if you need to say something because *you* are uncomfortable!

Corridor Cosy

This one can be tricky as you need to be in an enclosed area. The man needs to lean against a wall and needs to shuffle his way towards the floor until his feet are touching an opposing wall. The female should climb down on top of his legs, supporting her own weight. Her legs should be left dangling and she can begin thrusting.

This is a great one for adventurous and exciting sex!

Safety Tips

The male needs to make sure that he can support his partner's weight and that he isn't going to slip and fall to the floor completely. Likewise, the female should support her own weight as best she can to avoid potential injury.

Twister Stalemate

The female should begin by laying on her back with her legs apart. Her partner should kneel down on all fours in between her legs. The female should then lift herself up, wrapping her arms around his chest for support. She should then slowly bring up her legs so her feet are flat on the floor.

This is a great position for deep penetration and stimulating the G-spot!

Safety Tips

This position requires some upper body strength from the female. She should make sure to be holding on tightly to her partner as he thrusts.

The Spider

You should start by facing each other. The female should climb on to her partner's lap and allow penetration. Her legs should be bent on either side of him and the man should be doing the same. The female should lay back first, slowly followed by the man, until both heads are on the bed. Now, move slowly and calmly.

This is a great one for slow sex to enhance stimulation before trying to reach climax – a good one if you have a lot of time.

Safety Tips

This position requires penile flexibility, else there is a risk of the man straining his suspensory ligaments!

If you want to find out if the man's penis is flexible enough, have him stand against a wall. Pull his penis gradually down. If the penis is able to point directly down to the ground without causing pain then you should be fine to perform this position, but still be careful.

The woman should stay still when the man is initially penetrating her and guide the penis to the vagina. The woman should wait while he finds the most comfortable position and angle to thrust without injury.

Speed Bump

The female should lay on her stomach and spread her legs. The male should then enter from behind.

The benefit of this position is that things can heat up and speed up very quickly. It is a great position for getting a little rough or if you're having a quickie!

Safety Tips

This position can cause a lot of strain on the female's lower back, so make sure support is provided by using a pillow or cushion! Be sure to ask whether your partner is comfortable and not in any pain at any point and don't be ashamed if you need to say something because *you* are uncomfortable!

Triumph Arch

The man should sit down with his legs stretched out straight. The female should straddle him with her legs either side and kneel down over his penis. Once she has been penetrated, she can lean back until laying down on his legs.

This position can give the female a great orgasm and the male is able to stimulate her boobs and nipples during sex.

Safety Tips

This position requires penile flexibility, else there is a risk of the man straining his suspensory ligaments!

If you want to find out if the man's penis is flexible enough, have him stand against a wall. Pull his penis gradually down. If the penis is able to point directly down to the ground without causing pain then you should be fine to perform this position, but still be careful.

The woman should stay still when the man is initially penetrating her and guide the penis to the vagina. The woman should wait while he finds the most comfortable position and angle to thrust without injury.

The Propeller

The woman should lay on her back with her legs straight and together. The man should lie down on top, but facing down towards her feet. Once penetrated, the man should make small motions with his hips instead of thrusting.

This is a very difficult position and takes some practice to master!

Safety Tips

This position requires penile flexibility, else there is a risk of the man straining his suspensory ligaments!

If you want to find out if the man's penis is flexible enough, have him stand against a wall. Pull his penis gradually down. If the penis is able to point directly down to the ground without causing pain then you should be fine to perform this position, but still be careful.

The woman should stay still when the man is initially penetrating her and guide the penis to the vagina. The woman should wait while he finds the most comfortable position and angle to thrust without injury.

The Standing Wheelbarrow

For this position, begin in the doggy style position and have the female rest her forearms on some pillows. Her partner should kneel down behind her with one knee bent up to keep himself steady. Once he has penetrated, he should hold her feet and slowly lift her up as he stands.

This position is great if you are just experimenting and having a laugh! Otherwise, it is a bit difficult and isn't very well rated for sensation.

Safety Tips

The male should keep his knees slightly bent when thrusting. If either of you feel uncomfortable during the position then you should let the other know and try something else! This one isn't for you.

Sultry Saddle

In this position, the male lays down on his back with his legs bent and apart – the standard position when the male is on the bottom. The female should slide herself between his legs, almost at a right angle to his body. For support, one hand should be placed on his chest, the other on his leg.

This position relies on the female rocking back and forth until she can feel him hitting her G-spot. The great thing about this position is that the female is completely in control so is one of the better one if G-spot stimulation is what you need to reach an orgasm.

Safety Tips

This position can cause a lot of strain on the female's lower back, so make sure support is provided by using a pillow or cushion! Be sure to ask whether your partner is comfortable and not in any pain at any point and don't be ashamed if you need to say something because *you* are uncomfortable!

The Challenge

This is a difficult position (hence the name) and shouldn't be attempted unless you are confident and have tried lots of different positions before – it requires strength and flexibility.

The female should stand on a chair and bend her knees until in the sitting position. She should lean forward with her elbows on her knees. The male should then enter her from behind.

This one is hard to master.

Safety Tips

Make sure the chair is very sturdy and you have good footing. The male should support the female throughout and should have a firm hold of the woman's waist to keep her steady.

The Waterfall

The man should sit in a sturdy chair. The woman can then climb on top with her legs either side of him. She should lean back until her head is on the floor.

The clitoris is very accessible in this position so is great for stimulation during sex. There is also a lot of friction inside the vagina so this is a great all-rounder for reaching orgasm.

Safety Tips

This position requires penile flexibility, else there is a risk of the man straining his suspensory ligaments!

If you want to find out if the man's penis is flexible enough, have him stand against a wall. Pull his penis gradually down. If the penis is able to point directly down to the ground without causing pain then you should be fine to perform this position, but still be careful.

The woman should stay still when the man is initially penetrating her and guide the penis to the vagina. The woman should wait while he finds the most comfortable position and angle to thrust without injury.

A pillow should also be used on the floor to support and give comfort to the woman's head during sex.

Chapter 19: Sex for People with Mobility Challenges

It seems that a lot of people don't really care to talk much about sex and mobility issues. In a world in which taboos are getting knocked down faster than pins in a bowling alley that seems a little backward to me. Maybe that's because I've lived an experience of temporary disability and through that, have come to a fuller understanding of how that can play out in people's sex lives.

When I was scheduled for hip surgery, it hit me like a sledgehammer. I was too young. I was going to be completely helpless for as long as three weeks, using a walker. Then I'd be on a cane, learning how to walk with my new, bionic reality, all over again. I didn't relish the thought, but at the very least, I had a loving partner at my side to make the whole ordeal easier. When it finally came to attempting sex again, I learned what it was like to lose something, even if that loss was only temporary. This gave me a new respect and admiration for people who deal with disability and how that can impact their sexuality, every day of their lives.

When you go into the operating room, the last thing on your mind is sex. For one, you don't know if you'll ever wake up again. But once you get past that bit and you're on the mend – you remember that, yes – sex is good! You would like to have it again and soon. But what's a guy with a fresh hip replacement to do? It's counseled that you need at least six weeks prior to attempting sex again. In the meantime, there's always the Old Fashioned to keep you warm, not to mention the oral option, but your partner needs attention too.

For those with mobility issues, sex can be a challenge, but where there's a will there's a way, so this chapter's just for those of you who've either lost mobility temporarily, haven't had it for a while, or suffer from other physical challenges that make living out your sexuality a little more difficult than it is for most people.

The Ultimate Guide to Sex and Disability

This book is exactly what it says it is – a primer for those who live with a wide range of disabilities and challenges, but who continue to be enthusiastic about living out their sexuality. It's a comprehensive guide to sex, also, for those who suffer from conditions that cause them to suffer chronic pain (fibromyalgia), or chronic fatigue.

The book counsels the use of sex furniture, some of which is detailed in the previous chapter, like the wedge. This item can make sex a lot less physically stressful for those suffering from mobility issues, chronic pain, or both. While this may sound a little crazy, slings and swings are also a tremendous help for those who have physical limitations, or chronic pain. The weightlessness experienced in using these devices makes sex stress and pain-free operation. The Ultimate Guide enthusiastically counsels trying this solution when sex has taken a back seat to pain and/or disability and you're eager to get it back in your life. The Guide even gives "how-to" instructions on how to make your own sex sling. Now, there's a worthy project for you and a special friend!

Sex after Multiple Sclerosis

Almost all of us have a friend or family member who suffers from this disease. Maybe it's you. Maybe it's your partner. What we know, though, is that MS touches all our lives, with 2.5 million sufferers worldwide and almost half a million in the USA, alone. Every day, almost 200 new cases are diagnosed.

Mimi Mosher is an MS patient who helps other patients gets a handle on their sexual identities, following diagnosis. She believes that a healthy sexuality for MS people involves four crucial components, which are:

- Maintaining **confidence** in sexual identity is key for people with MS. A diagnosis can leave MS people feeling inadequate and insecure. Partners can certainly help with this side effect of the illness, as well as the family doctor.

- As I've tried to stress throughout this book, sex is a journey and it should be a fun one. That means that **exploration** part of the fun. For people with MS, whose nervous systems have been compromised by the disease, mobility issues may demand that partners are sensitive to the changes that can occur. Looking at sex from the perspective of intimacy (before gratification) can open the door to more satisfying sex for both partners. Instead of MS ruining the sex lives of couples in which one partner has the disease, it can broaden their horizons.

- As with any challenge that represents a change in mobility status, couples facing the challenge are called upon to **get creative**. Using lubricants that produce additional sensation, or employing vibrators and other means of enhanced stimulation can address a loss of sensation. Sex furniture can help, too. The key is an open discussion between partners about how you're going to meet the challenge and make it an exciting adventure you share together.

- All good sex demands **trial and error**. No one is born knowing how to be "good in bed". The challenge may be multiplied when MS is the third party in the bedroom, but that doesn't mean your curiosity should be stymied. It should, in fact, be stimulated by this new reality. Trying new things and letting go of those practices which no longer work for you is all part of what it means to be a loving couple, dedicated to one another's pleasure.

Men suffering from MS may have difficulty maintaining an erection, but this is not the end of the world, by any means. Problems with muscle cramps can also occur which make staying in the mood difficult. For this problem, the market is flooded with pharmaceutical aids that can help men maintain their erections. Also available are vacuum pumps and rings. These are also helpful for women partners with MS, who have lost some of their libido, but aren't willing to let their partners go without.

Pain and a loss of lubrication are also problems women with MS may suffer from. The same de-sensitizing lubricants used by men to delay ejaculation can be used by women to reduce discomfort when having intercourse. There are many such products available and they can all be used safely by women. Personal lubricants can help replace natural lubrication lost to MS and pave the way for pleasurable sex, without the discomfort generally associated with such loss.

Finally, spasticity is a common problem for people of both sexes, with MS. This can be exacerbated by orgasm. To help avoid the occurrence of muscle spasms, massage is indicated. The act of massage is one of the total, physical intimacy between partners. This activity can also be a substitute for intercourse at those times when it becomes difficult for one or both partners. By relaxing the muscles through prolonged massage (perhaps using a vibrator), partners can strengthen their bond and engage in a type of eroticism that is less demanding than more traditional methods of engaging in sexual activity. Massage is proven to reduce the occurrence of muscle spasms, thus making orgasm the pleasure it's supposed to be and not the problem it can be for people with MS.

No boundaries

Even my personal experience of temporary disability was difficult for me to absorb, as a man. Men suffer from a unique complex of insecurities centered on our sexuality that can make us extremely sensitivity to any perceived diminishment in our virility. Negative self-talk can take over, getting in the way of your sexuality and finally, killing it, as your sexual confidence takes a nosedive.

As I've written this book primarily for use by partners in long-term relationships and marriages, I'm going to address the same constituency here. A loving partner is a key ingredient for people with disabilities of any kind having a satisfying sex life. But a satisfying sex life is the birthright of all people and not only for those who have no physical challenges. That means that even people who are not partnered should able to live out their sexuality as fully as possible.

Whether this is done by autoerotic means (self-stimulation), or the use of sexual surrogates (people you can hire to assist you, sexually, dedicated to service to disabled people), it's the right of every living person to live out their sexuality.

Couples who support and love one another can find a way around any challenge or obstacle. In all the great love stories, love conquers all and that includes physical challenges like the loss of mobility, MS, chronic fatigue and chronic pain. When one of you is suffering, there is a world of help out there that you only have to look for and call on. Your life as a physically loving couple doesn't end with disability. It may, in fact, only be getting started.

Chapter 20: Other Ways of Pleasure

Everything that is new in the art of sexuality is well received by women. She wants to be amazed, and her emotionality is stimulated towards sensuality when unpublished games and fantasies are added to erotic relationships.

Routine and monotony are the great enemies to fight for lovers, as well as rigid attitudes and attachment to old patterns. If humor, imagination, and playful sense are introduced, the passion remains and new springs always sprout from it. This makes sure that sparks that ignite the bodies occur and cause more desire.

Fantasies for men begin with sight or touch, but for women, all of the five senses are alert and willing to take action and vibrate with joy in the arms of those who are capable of increasing the incitement and accompany her on that revealing route of sexuality creating new intimate sensations. On this inexhaustible space and road, deepening the feminine sensibility, she will find a companion always willing to go to the new places. The erotic fantasy of expanding exciting situations to reach the border of pleasure together is what she aims for.

The Game of the Roles

Creating a sexual relationship as if it were a stage or playing different roles is a way of reinventing pleasure. Inviting with your eyes without saying a word, inciting with the body adopting a special posture, or simply ignoring the other, acting as if you were alone, provokes passionate reactions.

She leans languidly as if she wanted to sleep. Her eyes are closed and she does not look at him or look for him, but something in her body seems to deny it, one thigh is shrunken and she sees pubic hair, the other leg is tense as it would be. Suddenly, he approaches and perceives the perfume that arises from the pubis, and he cannot resist the temptation to sink his face between the softness of her thighs and lick her until she abandons her lassitude and awakens all her erotic instincts with caress.

The Shared Bath

Underwater, everything glides naturally, the skin shines and it is easy to caress with the foam, play to make bubbles, provoke with the rubbing, to caress with the sponge as unintentionally, and move away. The water slides through her skin, he wraps her warm and perfumed body with his arms, but she turns her back and everything indicates that she resists and that she does not want more pleasure than the shared shower. However, he will try to seduce her with the force of his excitement. Kneeling down, he kisses the belly and her belly button and slowly descends down, licking with passion, until he feels it delivered and lost in the burning tide of desire he has awakened.

Erotic Dreams

Just as sexual fantasies appear during waking hours, during sleep, the world of the unconscious is still active and recreates erotic scenes. Sometimes, these are an enriched continuation of a reality that has been lived, but they can also be totally new because they come from hidden desires in the depths of the mind.

The sensual images of dreams have known or unknown protagonists, are plausible or incredible, which sometimes surprises the woman or even the mob by the bold look they present but since they contain so many complex and difficult-to-read symbols, it is impossible to draw certain conclusions about its meaning.

Most commonly, in dreams, repressed ideas or desires are expressed, whether by social conventions or prejudices, fears, or taboos. In this regard, she often dreams of multiple relationships, infidelities, homosexuality, and similar issues, which can be ghosts of women who, in reality, do not allow themselves to confess to themselves. However, do not get carried away by the guilt or contradiction that the dream images introduce, but try to incorporate the consciousness naturally. If something that is remembered when waking up can lead to reality and contributes to pleasure, it is positive to take advantage of it to enrich eroticism, as is done with fantasies, but if it generates anxiety or doubts, it is enough not to give it importance since Its meaning does not always respond to unspeakable desires.

Chapter 21: Preparations

Now that you've learned various lovemaking positions, it is important to learn the things you need to do before getting undressed. If you want to get maximum pleasure from sex, you must follow the instructions given here.

How to Prepare the Body

Before making love to your partner, you have to make sure that your body is fully prepared. This section of the book will teach you two important lessons about preparing your body for lovemaking.

The Smell of Your Breath

According to the Kama Sutra, body odor can dampen a person's sexual desires. If you'll combine it with bad breath, on the other hand, your partner's passion will be as cold as ice. Because of this, you have to make sure that your breath smells fresh. It's a good thing that different kinds and flavors of breath fresheners are available today.

People who have bad breath are usually unaware of their smelly situation. Sometimes, this lack of knowledge is caused by their partner's unwillingness to mention the problem. If you aren't confident with your breath, you must ask your partner to tell you the truth.

Taking a Bath Together

You may share the bathtub or take a shower together. By doing so, you will remove the dirt from your body and become ready for passionate lovemaking. You may also make love in the bathroom, though you have to be careful since the floor is slippery. Most people prefer to go to the bedroom than do "it" in the bathroom.

The "Hot Spots"

The brain is a sensitive sexual organ. In fact, many people claim that sex can be extremely boring if imagination is not involved. Regardless of their gender, people who are great in bed have an imaginative recognition of the human body's "hot spots." These hot spots are clinically known as "erogenous zones." To help you understand how these "spots" work, let's refer to these body parts as "pleasure spots," since they have the potential to heighten the sexual pleasures that the human body can achieve.

Obviously, the three major pleasure spots of the human body are:

- The skin

- The brain

- The genitals

By focusing on these pleasure zones, you can get your partner in the mood for lovemaking and boost his/her sexual desires. This section of the book will discuss two techniques that you can use on these hot spots: (1) kissing, and (2) touching.

> **Important Note:** Some people think that touching or kissing a person's feet is equivalent to foot fetishism. However, this isn't true. The feet have special reflex connections with the rest of a person's body. This is proven by the feet's importance in massage therapies.
>
> - *Butt*–Your partner's butt has lots of nerve endings. Thus, it offers great potential in heightening his/her sensual desires.

For some men, a woman's butt is more attractive than her breasts, particularly if the butt is highlighted by thin clothing. A woman's butt, just like her boobs, is naturally more pronounced than that of a man. Actually, it is the roundness and firmness of a woman's butt and breasts that attract men.

The buttocks of a woman serve three purposes:

- They attract men

- They enclose the woman's genitals

- They can be a source of sexual pleasure

A man can stimulate a woman's butt by squeezing, rubbing, slapping, kissing, or biting it gently. Some women like to do those things for their partner.

The Most Sensitive Parts of the Anus

Imagine a circle centered on the anus of your partner. Now, think of that circle as a clock, with the testicles or vagina acting as the 12 o'clock mark. The most sexually sensitive parts of his/her anus are the points at the 2 o'clock and 10 o'clock positions.

- *The Skin* –A human's skin has countless nerve endings that react to touches, pressure, and temperature changes. It is also considered as the largest organ of a human's body. That means you can exploit the natural sensitivity of your partner's skin in heightening his/her arousal.

- *The breasts* – the breasts of a woman play an important part in forming sexual attractions. Aside from attracting males, a woman's breasts are sensitive to touches and temperature changes. Thus, the breasts are one of the most important pleasure zones that must be stimulated during foreplay and lovemaking.

In general, the nipples and the areolae (i.e. the area of the breast that surrounds the nipple) are inherently sensitive to touches. Actually, some women attain orgasm when their nipples are stimulated orally or manually. Most women appreciate it when their partner rubs/kisses their nipples and gently squeezes their breasts. Many men, however, spend insufficient time stimulating their partner's breasts. The last statement holds true even for people who are aware of the breasts' potential in pleasing a woman sexually.

Important Note: The nipples are sensitive to touches and temperature changes. Sucking, kissing, and licking them gently can heighten a person's sexual desires. The sensations brought by skin-to-skin contact and the mouth's natural warmth can switch your partner's senses to overdrive.

How to Create the Right Mood

You also have to prepare the area where you and your partner will make love. According to the Kama Sutra, the feelings of the couple regarding their surroundings have a huge impact on their overall enjoyment. That means you have to decorate the room and make sure that it is conducive to passionate lovemaking. Here are the things that you can do to achieve the ideal atmosphere:

- Make sure that the area is cool when the weather is hot. When the weather is cold, on the other hand, ensure that the area is sufficiently warm (but not hot).

- Play some background music. Choose songs that can help you and your partner relax.

- Turn off your mobile phones and other gadgets that can produce noise. The last thing you want to happen is to get disturbed by a text message or phone call.

- Don't drink alcohol or eat too much. You will attain excellent performance in bed if you have a clear head and a satisfied (not full) tummy.

Conclusion

Sex is an important part of life and crucial for being in a fulfilling relationship. Whether you have a great sex life and just want to keep experimenting, or you're just starting to explore what makes you and your partner feel good, I hope this book has been a useful resource for you. Don't forget that this book is only a start. By opening up communication with your partner about sex, you can both continue to explore and grow sexually, figuring out how to have the most satisfying sexual relationship possible. Sex is for everyone, from flexible yogis to couch potatoes, so wink at your partner, shimmy out of your clothes, and start having fun!